FIFTY PLACES TO PRACTICE YOGA

BEFORE YOU DIE

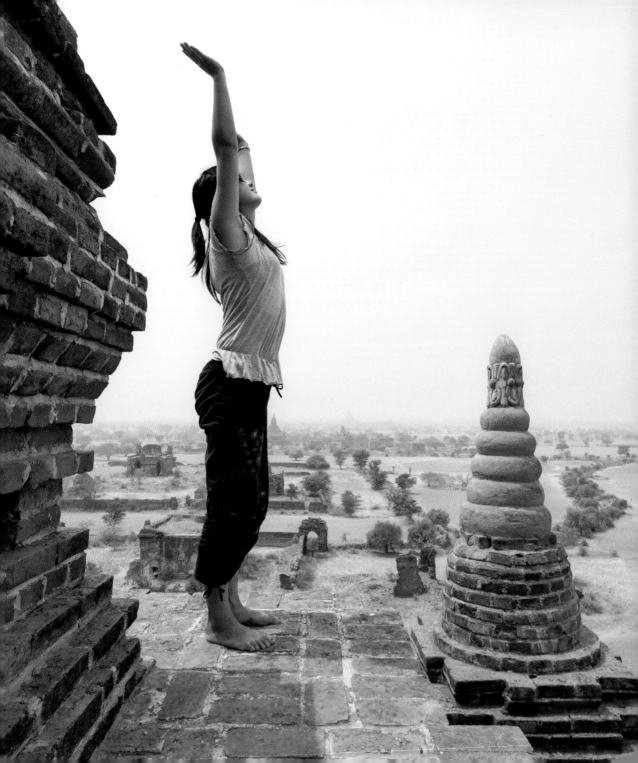

FIFTY PLACES TO PRACTICE

YOGA

BEFORE YOU DIE

**Yoga Experts Share
the World's Greatest Destinations**

Chris Santella *and* Diana Helmuth

FOREWORD BY STEWART GILCHRIST

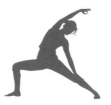

ABRAMS IMAGE

NEW YORK

This book is for our friends and family, who supported us writing through a difficult year of quarantine and helped us kindle dreams of seeing faraway places again.

Contents

Acknowledgments 9 / Foreword 11 / Introduction 13

THE DESTINATIONS

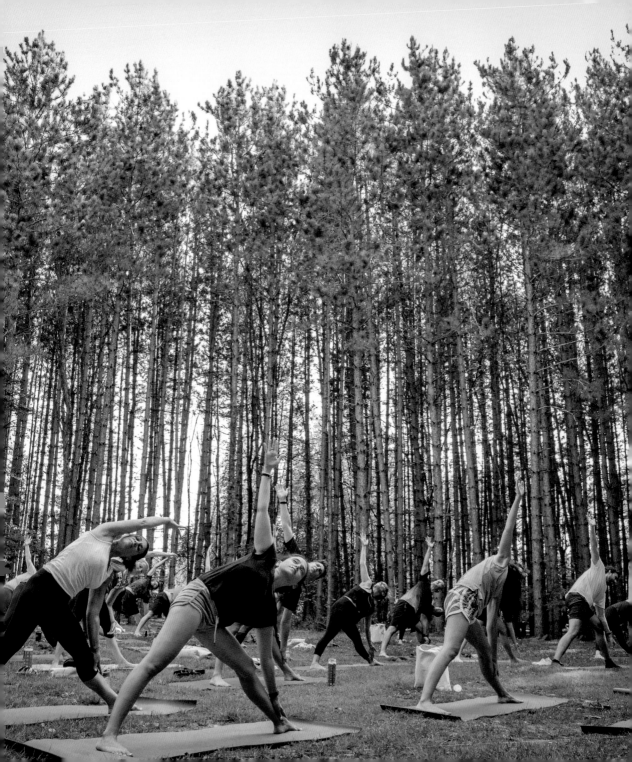

ACKNOWLEDGMENTS

This book would not have been possible without the assistance of the yoga teachers and spiritual leaders who shared their voices with us. To these men and women, we offer the most heartfelt thanks. We would also like to thank the editors Samantha Weiner, Elizabeth Broussard, and Annalea Manalili; designer Anna Christian; and copy editor Margaret Moore and proofreader Joy Sanchez Gillespie, who helped bring the book into being.

Diana would like to offer special thanks to Mitra Malek for kindly helping with introductions, her agent Danielle Svetcov, and Chris Santella for so warmly sharing the privilege of writing another volume in this special series. Special thanks to Justin Castilla and Joanna Robinson for their ongoing support, and her mother, who always encouraged her writing.

Chris would like to offer special thanks to his agent Stephanie Rostan, and his wife, Deidre, and daughters, Cassidy and Annabel, for their patience and unwavering support. And to Michael McDonough, whose yogic practice has long been an inspiration.

OPPOSITE:
Yogis enjoy a
midday flow
among the
tall trees at
Camp Walden
in Ontario.

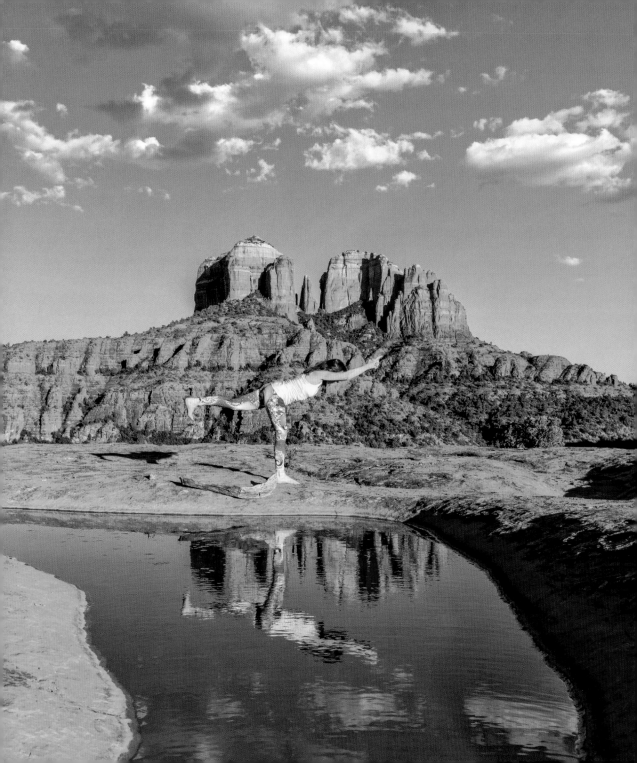

FOREWORD

"The times they are a-changin' . . ." When yoga resurfaced on the hippie scene back in the sixties, it was the time of Ginsberg, protests for civil rights and against the Vietnam War, LSD, Woodstock, and free love! Out of this renaissance grew a deep interest in the spiritual practices of ancient India, Tibet, and Southeast Asia: yoga, Buddhism, Ayurveda, tantra, devotional music, and much more.

These pioneers of modern yoga practiced in youth centers, church halls, community centers, parks, and beaches. In fact, anywhere they could light incense, chant mantra, and do asana and meditate, they would. The Beatles, the Bhagavad Gita, Ravi Shankar, B. K. S. Iyengar, Hare Krishnas, Tibet, and Zen Buddhists all became part of everyday life as yoga started to find a foothold in America and the West.

Fifty years later, yogaprenueurs have created a billion-dollar industry of studios, retreats, clothing, mats and props, online tuition forums, and a plethora of disposable accessories that only a consumer culture like ours could possibly dream up. The ethics for some have gone by the wayside, the dharma altered by material attachment.

But despite all the hype, the desire to expand one's practice, and to explore the world through yoga, persists.

The diversity of places to practice range now from the splendor of high-end retreats across the globe, such as Ananda Spa outside Rishikesh, to a quiet beach in Kerala to a wooden cabin in Norway. *Fifty Places to Practice Yoga Before You Die* hopefully will assist you in finding your own favorite and niche places to practice, whatever your chosen path to yoga.

—Stewart Gilchrist
Senior registered yoga teacher, Yoga Alliance Professionals, UK

OPPOSITE:
The warm desert rocks of Sedona create a welcoming environment for yogis to connect with the earth.

11

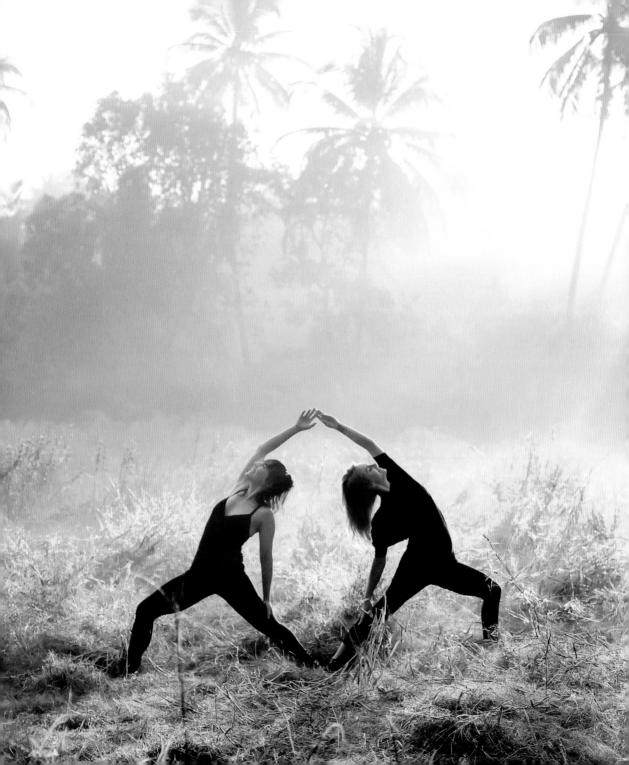

INTRODUCTION

According to Mitra Malek, a former *Yoga Journal* editor, "There are so many types of yoga, and they all have the same ultimate aspiration: enlightenment. Yoga, at its core, is both an acceptance and a freedom of the self. A yoga mat is an incredibly safe space to go inward, to try different things, to risk feeling uncomfortable, to risk feeling confident. It's a safe space to explore yourself and practice self-acceptance. There's no end goal in yoga except to keep moving toward an aspiration."

Yoga originated in the Indus Valley of India nearly five thousand years ago. The word is derived from the Sanskrit root *yuj*, meaning "to join" or "to unite." In its earliest incarnation, yoga was considered a spiritual discipline, its practice leading to the union of individual consciousness with universal consciousness, resulting in harmony between the mind and body, man and nature. Shiva, one of the principal deities of Hinduism, is considered the first yogi (or Adiyogi) and guru. It's believed that Shiva shared his profound knowledge with the seven sages (or Saptarishi) on the banks of lake Kantisarovar in the Himalayas, and this wisdom was carried far and wide, to Asia, Northern Africa, the Middle East, and South America.

As time passed, the practice of yoga evolved. The period between 500 BCE and 800 CE is considered India's classical period. Some of yoga's most revered texts were developed during this time, including the Bhagavad Gita, which presented the tenets of gyana, bhakti, and karma yoga. The post-classical period (800 CE to 1,700 CE) saw the birth of hatha yoga, thanks to teachers like Matsyendranatha, Cauranginatha, Gheranda, and Shrinivasa Bhatt. The next two hundred years are considered the modern period, when raja yoga developed and hatha yoga continued to flourish.

Yoga began to reach the West in the late nineteenth century—both as a spiritual practice and an exercise system for the preservation, maintenance, and promotion of health. Swami Vivekananda first spoke about yoga to Americans in 1893 at the Parliament of World's Religions in Chicago, and Paramahansa Yogananda founded the first yoga institutions in Los Angeles in the 1920s. As the century progressed, so did the world's journey along this path to self-acceptance and inner peace, paved with a little sweat. The twentieth century saw the rise of Swami Vishnudevananda, guru to the Beatles and father of the first yoga teacher training courses in the West; B. K. S. Iyengar, father of Iyengar yoga and

OPPOSITE:
Morning sun filters through palm trees along the Goan coast, a popular yoga vacation destination in India.

author of the foremost book on yoga anatomy; and Sri K. Pattabhi Jois, the founder of ashtanga yoga and the spiritual parent of the power yoga found on nearly every street corner of each major city in the world today. (The Beatles' visit to Rishikesh in 1968 to study transcendental meditation with Maharishi Mahesh Yogi, encouraged by George Harrison, may have done more to popularize yogic practices in the West than any other event.)

From calm, meditative yin yoga to gymnastic AcroYoga—and every style in between—yoga is now available on every continent to virtually everybody on earth, and it shows no signs of stopping.

The presence of yoga across the globe has presented practitioners with ample opportunity to see and be inspired by how different societies integrate yoga into their culture; it is wanderlust with a mission. Most yogis agree that yoga is ultimately a mind-set that transforms your relationship to your outside environment and to yourself, rather than an activity dependent on your environment. By following the eight-limbed path, of which *asana* (physical posture practice) is just once branch, dedicated yogis seek to weave harmony between their body, mind, and spirit, and develop a peace that stays with them wherever they are. However, although such journeys of self-inquiry can be achieved anywhere, it often requires breaking out of our routines and leaving our familiar environments behind to move us forward. This is where the magic of travel meets the grounding practice of yoga.

And that's what inspired us to write *Fifty Places to Practice Yoga Before You Die*.

So what makes a destination a place to practice yoga before you die? For some, it may be an opportunity to learn at the feet of a celebrated teacher. For others, a chance to connect with the elements in their practice, or reconnect with old friends. One thing was certain: We knew that we were not the people to assemble such a list. So we followed a recipe that worked well in the first sixteen Fifty Places books. We interviewed a host of people closely connected with the yoga world and asked them to share some of their favorite experiences.

In this book you will find yogis from around the world sharing their stories of successful crossings of life's rough passages, always with yoga as the path. Some are venerated masters of specific lineages (such as renowned yin master Josh Summers, or R. Alexander Medin, one of only thirty-five people certified by Sri K. Pattabhi Jois to teach ashtanga); some are rulebreakers and groundshakers (such as London's legendary Stewart Gilchrist or Drunk Yoga's founder, Eli Walker); and others are certified professional counselors and

14

therapists (such as life coach Rachel Wainwright and Dr. Barbara Vacarr, psychologist and director of Kripalu). Some are newer to their practice, and some have been practicing since they could walk. All have chosen to speak about these locations based on personal, profound memories, or the savoring of secret gems that have nourished them in ways no other simple "vacation" has. While the book collects fifty great venues, it by no means attempts to rank the places discussed. Such ranking is, of course, largely subjective. Instead, consider this a sample of the natural world and its wonders that have informed the metaphysical journey for these leaders.

Whether you seek to pilgrimage to the sacred waters of the Ganges in Rishikesh, India; ground into Mountain Pose on the slopes of Haines, Alaska; flow into Mermaid Pose on the coastline of Popoyo, Nicaragua; or waddle into Whale Pose next to the penguins of Antarctica, there is a yoga destination for you.

We hope that the stories herein will inspire you to find your reset button, enjoy your inner journey, and enhance your practice—and that what you discover out there can be something you bring home forever.

NEXT PAGE: Mysuru is considered the birthplace of ashtanga yoga.

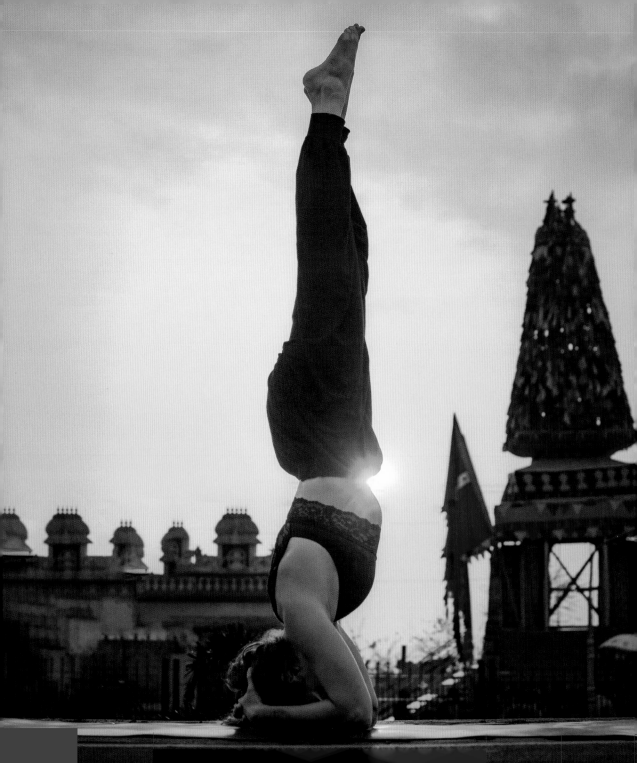

The Destinations

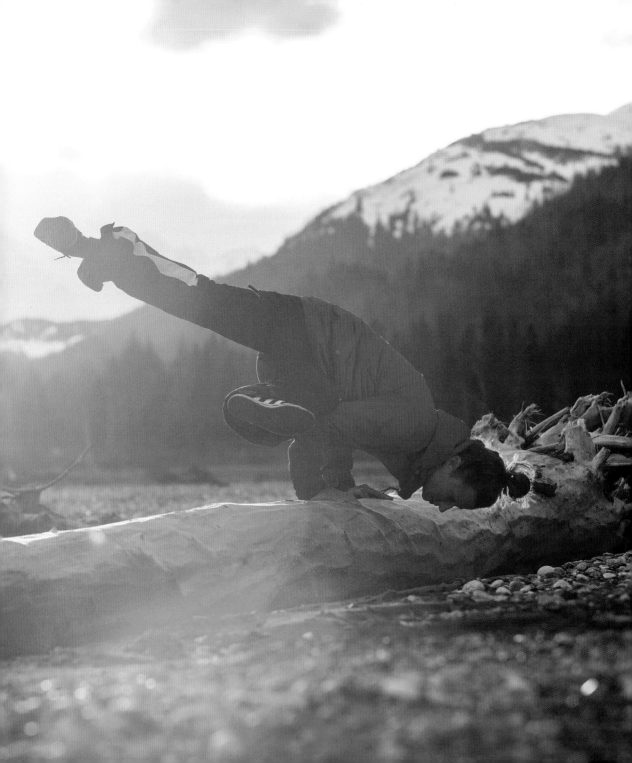

HAINES

RECOMMENDED BY **Sarana Miller**

"I think John Muir once said something like 'Don't let your young people go to Alaska because they'll never come home,'" Sarana Miller ventured. "I like to say, 'Don't let your yogis come to Alaska, or they'll never come home.'"

America's northernmost state—famous for sub-freezing winds, ten-foot grizzly bears, and roiling seas that contain "the Deadliest Catch"—might not strike most people as the ideal place to practice the world's most calming sport. "When I first went up there, it was at the recommendation of a man I met at Wilbur Hot Springs, in Northern California, where I was teaching at the time," Sarana recalled. "He said, 'You need to come check out Alaska.' I said, 'Why? What's in Alaska?' He eventually convinced me, and I went up to Haines, just to see what the fuss was about. I got off the plane, got into the nature, and almost immediately realized that I was exhausted. I was exhausted from teaching yoga in the San Francisco Bay Area, from fourteen classes a week. I was exhausted from running around trying to fit as much into my life as I could. And suddenly, here I was, surrounded by moss, ferns, berries, present to this abundance I didn't know my body was missing."

Often named one of the top-ten places to live in America, Haines is far from an unforgiving Arctic tundra. In fact, it's a temperate rainforest. Only accessible by a once-daily 4.5-hour ferry (that's after your connecting flights to Juneau), visitors who can tolerate the multiple-leg voyage will find themselves greeted by a Disney-esque landscape of woodland wonder— snow-frosted peaks, lush greenery, and shimmering lakes.

Hooked, Sarana started teaching locals, eventually bringing up other yogis who had never heard of the hidden gems that awaited in the north. "I love to take people to remote, beautiful places, offline and into beauty," said Sarana. "We set up the retreat center nestled along the Chilkat River, where the forest meets the ocean. We are right on the water,

OPPOSITE:
The forested mountains and cool riverbanks of Haines are a yogi's paradise in the spring and summer.

19

surrounded on all sides by three-thousand-foot mountains. It's rustic and extremely private . . . just a small grouping of yurts and a wooden meditation lodge. You get there by walking down through the forest, until you come upon the main yurt. Nearby is the temple. It's a timber frame mortise and tenon structure, built completely without nails. The entire building is essentially windows. You are surrounded by trees and green.

"In the morning, we serve chai, and then we'll come together in silence to do our meditation at the timber frame lodge. We're right on the water with a crackling wood fire going. I do a short talk of intention. Then we do a kirtan together and begin a silent meditation. You can only hear the water and the fire. Then, still in silence, we come back together and walk to the yoga yurt, and I lead a two-hour active asana. After that it's lunch in the lodge and then free time," Sarana described. In Haines, that means "frolicking in waist-high grass, picking berries off the vines, watching the salmon coming in, foraging for chanterelle mushrooms, and soaking up the energy of the spruce trees." Visitors can also marvel at the third most variable changing tide in the world. "It goes WAY out and then WAY in. It's right next to you at the meditation building, and then it's way out by the time you have opened your eyes."

To learn more about the early human inhabitants of Haines, you can visit the nearby First Nations village of Klukwan, which roughly translates to "forever village." Klukwan is the last of the five Chilkat villages that were in the area before 1900. The Chilkat people host many courses built around traditional knowledge, languages, and original arts.

Above all, though, Haines is a hiker's paradise. "The hiking trails are magnificent," Sarana enthused. "Mount Riley is right next to us. We hike up to the top and get a 360-degree panoramic view of the Deishú peninsula. Then you can climb back down and jump into the lake. I love Riley, but we also do another hike called 'chilly ridge' on Mount Ripinski. You get on the trail and hike four thousand feet, straight up from sea level. It's past the tree line, and then you're just among heather. You're above the world. It's quite arduous. This is something I wouldn't recommend doing on a yoga day, but it's incredible. You're at the top of the world, surrounded by flowers, and in August you can basically eat your way up, picking blueberries, salmonberries, watermelon berries." Animal lovers might be pleased to know that black bears, wolves, and even grizzlies call this area home—but intimate encounters with these bigger fauna are fortunately unlikely.

"Getting everyone to arrive in the morning in silence is so potent," Sarana reflected. "It's a pregnant quiet, to have a whole 1- to 1.5-hour of silence, facing the water and the glaciers, just soaking in the beauty and breathing. It's incredibly touching for your own spirit. There's a deep coming home, a realization that we're here to support each other. Finding our own inner stillness, but together, with the group. The beauty around us creates this alchemical oven for transformation.

"I've traveled all over the world, and I have to say that Alaska is the most nourishing place I've ever found, not just because of the land, but the people. Alaskans are incredibly generous with their time and resources. It shows from not only how they treat strangers, but also how they treat their dogs and their gardens. They're incredibly capable and have a huge generosity of spirit. We need that in our world."

SARANA MILLER was born and raised at California's Wilbur Hot Springs and is a graduate of the Piedmont Yoga Advanced Studies Program and the Forrest Yoga Teacher Training Program. Her yoga training is based on Iyengar and Forrest yoga traditions. She is a faculty instructor at *Yoga Journal* and teaches at the prestigious Claremont Hotel in Oakland, California, as well as at her own home studio. Her love of yoga was born at the Esalen Institute in 1997, where she continues to assist and teach with Thomas Fortel, her mentor and dear friend. She has also studied kirtan with Jai Uttal and classical Indian voice in India. She leads kirtans in the San Francisco Bay Area and is very thankful to be able to share this practice with others.

If You Go

▶ **Getting There**: Most people fly into Juneau, via Seattle or directly, on Delta (800-221-1212; delta.com) and Alaska Airlines (800-654-5669; alaskaair.com). From Juneau, a ferry can take you the hour trip to Haines.

▶ **Best Time to Visit**: May through mid-August brings the fairest weather, and the summer generally stays cool; under 70 degrees Fahrenheit is the daily high in July (with nineteen hours of sunshine on the summer solstice). Most of the winter is subfreezing, but full of powder for winter-sports lovers.

▶ **Accommodations**: The Chilkat Retreat Center is bookable at chilkatinletretreat.com. Beyond the summer forest, the Haines Visitor Center offers year-round accommodation options at visithaines.com.

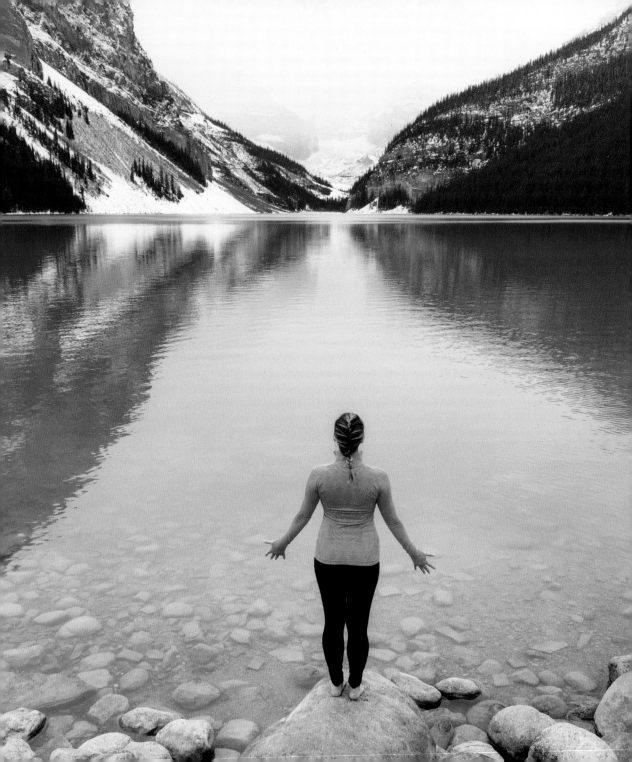

LAKE LOUISE

RECOMMENDED BY **Davina Bernard**

Banff National Park encompasses 2,564 square miles of amazingly pristine valleys, meadows, and mountains along the southern border between Alberta and British Columbia. The park—home to over a thousand glaciers and iconic Canadian Rockies creatures like grizzly bears, mountain goats, and wolves—is also home to two first-class resort properties, Fairmont Chateau Lake Louise and Fairmont Banff Springs.

"We like to say that visitors to Banff National Park go to Fairmont Banff Springs to visit the incredible spa, eat great food, and shop," Davina Bernard began. "They come to the Fairmont Chateau Lake Louise to be able to step out the door into nature. There's a magic here. You feel like you're in the middle of a postcard. It's hard to verbalize why it feels so good here, but there's a profound energy shift as you sit by the lake. The mountains are so old, and they seem to hug you. The old-growth pines here are covered in a moss known as old man's beard, which only grows where the air is completely pure. The hotel's water comes from the lake, which is fed by Victoria Glacier. Between showering and drinking that water, Lake Louise becomes part of you. Some feel that the Lake Louise area is one of the earth's major vortex spots. Whether it's that energy or just the natural beauty of the place, Lake Louise is a wonderful spot to re-center and have a transformational wellness experience."

That the Chateau and Banff Springs exist in the national park is thanks in large part to the Canadian Pacific Railway and the laws of supply and demand; the railroad created a supply of westbound train seats, and the hope was that some recreational centers would create a demand. The railway did not underestimate Banff's appeal. "The Banff Springs Hotel was built around the hot springs that bubbled up there to appeal to the spa culture," offered guide Michael Vincent, who works with Chateau Lake Louise's Mountain

OPPOSITE:
The turquoise
waters of
Lake Louise
provide
a stunning
backdrop for
restorative
experiences.

Adventure Program. "The original structure at Lake Louise—a log chalet with two bedrooms—was built for people interested in mountaineering. In 1899, several professional Swiss mountain guides were hired and brought to Lake Louise to help guests climb the surrounding mountains." The initial log cabin at Lake Louise burned to the ground, eventually giving way to the monolithic lodge that sits on what the Stoney Nakota First Nations people called Lake of Little Fishes. (Lake Louise's incredible turquoise color, incidentally, is the result of rock flour that's carried in the glacial melt that feeds the lake. Sunlight reflecting off the mineral particles refracts blue and green.)

Lake Louise's wellness program is the fruit, in some ways, of Davina's career journey. "I was born near Jasper (just north of Banff), and then moved to Ontario at the age of ten, though I always considered myself a mountain person," she continued. "I came to work for Fairmont right out of college and worked in the corporate office for ten years. I came out to Lake Louise almost a decade ago. My background had been in marketing and revenue management, but I shifted to product development and special events. In this role, I helped introduce mindfulness weekends, with yoga, lifestyle discussions, and great food. The idea was well received, and now the retreats are a regular part of the Lake Louise offering."

The retreats at Lake Louise are designed for people who are new to yoga. "It's an entry-level kind of program," Davina described. "For many attendees, they came across the notion of increased wellness somewhere. It was intriguing, but also scary and new. We offer a program where you're introduced to new ideas, but everything else in your life stays the same with all of the luxury services you expect from Fairmont."

Davina described how a Lake Louise wellness day generally unfolds. "The first full day begins with an hour and a half yoga session, a flow to get your body moving and focusing on the fundamentals. Morning yoga is followed by a buffet breakfast with almost endless options—the pumpkin bread and croissant French toasts are favorites. Breakfast is followed by an information session with our guest leader. We've attracted a number of notable leaders in the past, including Tracey Delfs, Shannon Kaiser, Elizabeth Trinkaus, Sophie Uliano, and many others. After lunch, participants have three hours on their own. Some will opt to visit the spa; others may wish to get outside. During our March/April sessions, that might mean snowshoeing or skating on Lake Louise; in October/November, perhaps a guided nature walk to see the surrounding mountains in the autumnal glory. We'll come together again for a gentle yoga and meditation session before dinner." Guests who visit Lake Louise in the heart of winter to ski, or in the summer to hike and canoe, have the option to squeeze in a yoga class, as instructors are present year-round. "During the summer, an evening stretch class is offered on the boathouse dock," Davina added, "so you're able to practice above the lake.

"Many of our guests are women over the age of forty-five, and they come on their own," Davina shared. "They haven't really done something like this before and are searching for something to make their life fuller, for ways to live the best life. They are very apprehensive the first night. But as they start to move together in the yoga practice, they begin to laugh. Many women bond over movement and food, and they leave having formed strong friendships. At the end of a retreat, we like to gather the group outside the chateau for a photo. The mountains surrounding the lake reflect the strength that they've built.

"It's beautiful to behold."

DAVINA BERNARD has worked in a number of roles during her career at Fairmont Hotels & Resorts. Her career ultimately led her to the path of yoga, mindfulness, and overall wellness in both her personal and professional lives. Organizing wellness retreats at Chateau Lake Louise since 2011 ignited a fire of mindfulness that took her to Plum Village in France to study with Thich Nhat Hanh's sangha. Making sure that Lake Louise's wellness guests have incredible, life-changing experiences is her passion.

If You Go

▶ **Getting There**: Banff National Park begins approximately sixty miles west of Calgary, Alberta; Lake Louise is another forty-odd miles from the park entrance. Calgary is served by many major carriers, including Air Canada (888-247-2262; aircanada.com); Alaska Airlines (800-252-7522; alaskaair.com); and Delta (800-221-1212; delta.com).

▶ **Best Time to Visit**: Wellness retreats are held in March/April and October/November. Yoga classes are available throughout the year.

▶ **Accommodations**: The Fairmont Chateau Lake Louise (403-522-3511; fairmont.com/lake-louise) has 539 guest rooms overlooking the lake or the mountains of Banff National Park. Specifics about upcoming wellness retreats are highlighted at lakelouisewellness.com.

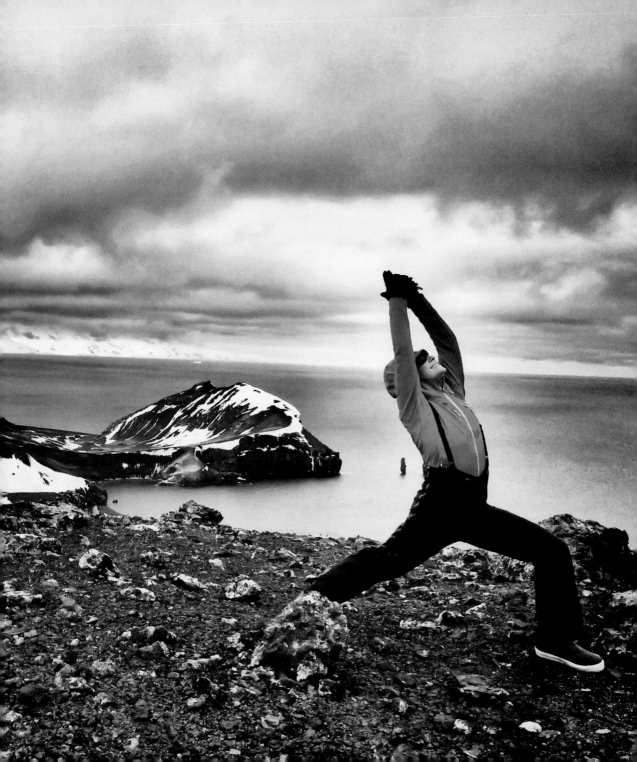

ANTARCTIC PENINSULA

RECOMMENDED BY **Elly MacDonald**

"There's something that happens in Antarctica," Elly MacDonald opined. "It has that last-frontier feeling. "When you're there, you realize how precious the world is, and how small we are in comparison."

For much of the year, Antarctica is not among the world's most welcoming places. This is evidenced by the lack of indigenous people on the continent, despite the fact that Antarctica encompasses over fourteen million square miles, roughly one and a half times the size of the United States! (A contingent of five thousand scientists from the twenty-seven nations that are signatories of the Antarctic Treaty maintain a year-round presence on the continent; another forty thousand or so tourists visit each season.) A great majority of the landmass—an estimated 98 percent—consists of ice and snow that has an average thickness of seven thousand feet; scientists believe that up to 70 percent of the world's fresh water is contained here. Put another way: If the ice stored in Antarctica were to melt, the world's oceans would rise two hundred feet. The continent is quite mountainous, with peaks (like Vinson Massif) over sixteen thousand feet. In the summer (December through March), the freeze recedes, and a brief window opens for sailing to the more northerly portions of Antarctica, like the Antarctic Peninsula.

Elly joined Quark Expeditions in 2016 to establish a yoga program on the company's Antarctic expeditions, which are conducted on ships built to withstand the challenging conditions encountered on the voyage south from Cape Horn across the Drake Passage. Waves that can reach heights of sixty-five feet prompted her to develop a special program for travel days. "Think low to the ground!" she explained. "Many of the poses are done seated or on our backs. It's a lot of core work, in addition to the core work you're already doing to stay steady on a moving ship. Everyone appreciates this, as the food is delicious

OPPOSITE:

Most of the yoga
on Antarctic
expeditions
occurs on the
ship, but some
will take their
practice to shore.

on the ship. And the deep stretches are great for limbering you up for hiking, snowshoeing, cross-country skiing, mountaineering, kayaking, or Zodiac cruising. On the first day at sea, I have a briefing in the lounge area. I ask everyone to get seated on the ground. If they're uncomfortable, the yoga program may not be for them, although I do try to make it accessible to everyone."

It's almost five hundred miles from Cape Horn to the Shetland Islands, at the northern tip of the continent of Antarctica. As you push beyond the Shetlands, you'll pass through alleys of icebergs—cracking, rolling, with massive chunks calving off—and the wildness of the seventh continent will begin to unfold. "Some guests are a little anxious during the crossing," Elly continued. "Yoga is a great way to bring people together and create a calm environment. Our first class is generally between six and seven A.M., and our room can accommodate up to twenty-two people. This is a shorter class, usually forty-five minutes. Depending on conditions, we may do a longer class in the late afternoon or evening." When you reach Antarctica, yoga sessions are scheduled around the excursions that enable guests to get close to the continent's incredible animal life—massive rookeries of penguins, colonies of seals, and pods of various whales (blue, bowhead, right, humpback, minke, and gray) that migrate here to feed on an abundance of krill. Excursions are conducted via Zodiac boat, hiking, and kayaking.

"The experiences we have on excursions are life-changing," Elly enthused. "I love whales, and the whale sightings I've had the last five years have been incredible, even spiritual. This past season, I was in a Zodiac with guests when a pod of humpbacks came around the raft. They were so curious and happy, slapping their fins and spyhopping right beside the boat for long periods. [Spyhopping is a behavior where the whale keeps its head out of the water to observe goings-on.] At times, we could see the whale's entire body, just underneath the boat. It was overwhelming and remains vivid in my memory. I also have been able to watch leopard seals on the hunt. [These predators, identified by their slightly reptilian head and a white throat that's decorated with black spots, are the only seal that will attack and devour other seals; a facial expression that might be likened to a crooked smile enhances their sinister reputation.] They look harmless when they're resting on the ice, but it's another story when they're swimming and hunting. The first time I watched a hunt, the seal caught a penguin. I thought I'd never want to witness this, but after I did, I had a greater appreciation of the circle of life. As the seal was feeding on the penguin carcass, all the seabirds began coming in for their share. Life is hard in

Antarctica. This is also evident around the penguin colonies, where brown skuas are always waiting to steal away chicks."

Elly usually conducts her yoga classes after the first excursion of the day. If the weather gods permit, sometimes she and her group can take their mats outside. "Once in a while, we get to do yoga on land, though it's not often," she said. "It has to be the perfect day, and we have to be in an area where there's enough space and no wildlife nearby. If it's a warmer day, we can do a yoga class on the outer deck. There have been times when we're out there and a pod of whales or orcas come by. It's a very emotional moment. Some people have the happiness cry."

ELLY MACDONALD grew up on the shores of Lake Erie, Canada, where she gained an appreciation for water and earth at an early age. She has ventured to many places around the world, expanding her knowledge and experiences with several cultures. Elly's passion and main source of connection is yoga. She has been teaching and studying different styles and levels of this practice for fifteen years, giving her a greater awareness of presence and gratitude. She has a keen interest in various healing modalities and wellness and plans to share her energy and excitement with all she encounters. Elly also has a passion for the world's polar regions. Guiding guests on land and sea has been tremendously rewarding. Toronto, Canada, is Elly's home base, where she is continually learning from all her students and looking for the next adventure.

If You Go

► **Getting There**: Most groups gather in Buenos Aires (which is served by most major carriers. From there, you'll fly to Ushuaia and join a boat to sail south. Ushuaia is served by several carriers, including Aerolíneas Argentinas (aerolineas.com.ar) and LATAM Airlines (866-435-9526; latam.com).

► **Best Time to Visit**: Expeditions to Antarctica are offered from November through March.

► **Accommodations**: The trip described above is orchestrated by Quark Expeditions (888-979-4073; quarkexpeditions.com).

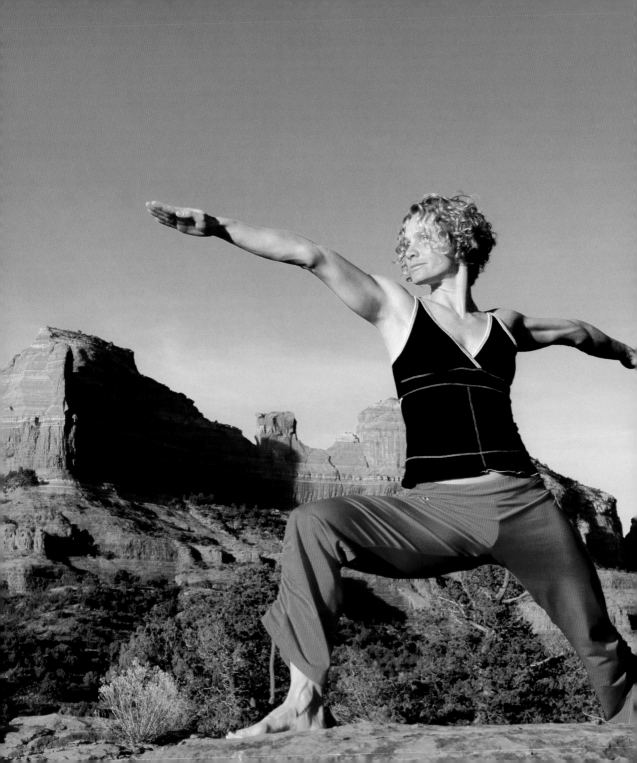

SEDONA

RECOMMENDED BY **Yogi Blair Darby**

The red-hued desert oasis known as Sedona has long been a haven for nature-lovers, New Age iconoclasts, and spiritual searchers. "It is the only place like it on earth," began Yogi Blair. "I came here initially for a workshop on the Tree of Life. At the time, I was splitting my time between Phoenix and Cottonwood. I was driving a lot, feeling somewhat disconnected. My dad kept telling me 'You gotta come check out Sedona,' and I thought, *What's Sedona, and what does Dad know?* Then I arrived, and I saw the red rocks, and immediately my heart was just pulled."

Arizona's famously mystic city is located at the base of the Mogollon Rim, the southwestern border of America's arid Colorado Plateau. Over millions of years, erosion has gradually moved the rim northward out of the earth's crust, leaving behind some of the most picturesque canyons and buttes found anywhere in the world, often in beguiling formations painted by Mother Nature in rich pink and red hues. Not to be confused with a barren desert, from all this red rock bursts forth cypress and ash trees, as well as cliffrose and sage shrubs, fed by numerous streams and creeks burbling out of the hillsides and converging into rivers and pool throughout the valleys.

Subsequently, Sedona is a nature-lover's dream come true. Hundreds of hiking trails and dirt roads weave through the towering red rocks, leading to heavenly vistas or green, shaded valleys, with creeks beckoning you for a dip. For a true immersion in crimson, you can day trip or hire a tour out to Red Rock State Park and gape at the skyscraper-esque formations that glow in the sunset. Those interested in Native American history and way of life before colonization can visit the Native American Palatki Heritage Site, or charter a Jeep tour to the Palatki and Honanki cliff dwellings for an intimate viewing of thousand-year-old petroglyphs.

OPPOSITE: Sedona offers numerous opportunities to practice outside and connect with the unique geology of the area.

31

"One of my favorite things to do," enthused Blair, "is take people through the mystical red rocks on a hike, until we come upon an epic spot, maybe at the top of a plateau, or overlooking a creek, whereupon we practice yoga. We also do affirmations, meditations, breathing exercises, Qi Gong—it's a perfect space for all of it. The potential for movement here is so strong, working with the energies of the rocks and the vortexes. You look at the plants, savoring all the sensations around you. The time goes by so fast when you're outside. We don't rush. It's good to soak up your surroundings."

Beyond its dreamy geologic formations, Sedona's most famous (or infamous) pull might be its vortexes. "The vortexes swirl you into a cotton-candy sweet place in your heart," Blair described. "They're a mix of the Tasmanian devil, Madonna, Mahatma Gandhi, and Muhammad Ali." According to some, Sedona's energy vortexes are caused by the magnetic field around the earth bumping up against a layer of quartzite that rests unassumingly 1,500 feet below Sedona's surface, spreading out for an entire mile in all directions. "It's a magical enchanted bling-bling underworld down there," Blair said with a smile. "The crystal is so powerful that it energetically shatters the magnetic field, creating the vortexes.

"But it's not just the vortexes that make Sedona so special," explained Blair. "It's the ley lines: concentric energy lines that run across the earth and create energy highways that run through the planet. One of them runs right through Sedona. So, the vortexes, mixed with the iron oxide and quartzite in the earth, and then the ley lines, all work together to create a yummy tossed salad of synergistic symphonies that you can feel when you're here. This isn't the only place on earth where you can see these forces, but those four forces together? This is exclusive to Sedona."

The forces have made Sedona a famous international hub of alternative healers, avant-garde spiritual workshops, holistic medicine, New Age philosophy, and, of course, yoga, including the massive, thousand-plus-bodies-strong Sedona Yoga Festival that takes place every March. It has also given rise to what might be America's most prominent crystal and gemstone scene. "Some people come to Sedona just to charge their crystals," Blair explained. "This could be to help them find peace in the mystic chaos or enhance their intuition. Some people simply infuse them with the experience of Sedona, so they can take it home with them.

"For those who can feel this convergence, this energy, it can take you by surprise," continued Blair. "You feel the cosmic internet all the time out here, but sometimes it really sneaks up on you. That could be after dancing, or a breathing exercise, or a loving moment, or whatever. Sometimes it shows up when you least expect it. One day, I was doing a meditation with my friend out at Cathedral Rock, and I felt this jolt. We both looked at each other at the same time like 'Wow, did you feel that?'

"It's par for the course that some people will say they want to feel the energy, but then they don't," noted Blair. "Sedona energy amplifies the good and the bad. If you're not dealing with your bad stuff, don't come. It can put the mousetrap on your butt. But for most folks, after they spend a few days clearing their minds, they can really open up.

"I had some challenging moments when I first moved here," concluded Blair, "but using the energy here to amplify my intentions and build the life I wanted to create, it's great. I came from a place of struggle. But I used the power and beauty of Sedona to create a new, intentional life."

YOGI BLAIR DARBY spent his entire life in the beach town of Venice, California, before he, his girlfriend, and his son packed up and moved to the beautiful red-rock-adorned area of Sedona, where his passion for energies and yoga would reach new and unexpected heights. Though well practiced in a variety of yoga methods, in both modern and traditional practices, Blair attributes his success to his ability to help others see Sedona through a whole new lens. A yoga and Qi Gong teacher, he incorporates new practices and teachings to his popular yoga hiking experiences, including hiking, integrating color and sound therapy, and utilizing crystal photonic light therapy's beneficial healing properties.

If You Go

▶ **Getting There**: Sedona's closest airport is Flagstaff Airport, although its small size is not served by many carriers. Phoenix International Airport, served by American Airlines (800-433-7300; aa.com) and Southwest (800-435-9792; southwest.com), is an easier bet. Most folks rent a car for the two-hour ride, but shuttles can also be chartered.

▶ **Best Time to Visit**: The Sedona Yoga Festival typically takes place in March, and most of spring sees wonderful blooms across the mountainsides.

▶ **Accommodations**: The Sedona Tourism Board (sedona.net) lists a variety of accommodations, from upscale hotel chains to rustic cabins.

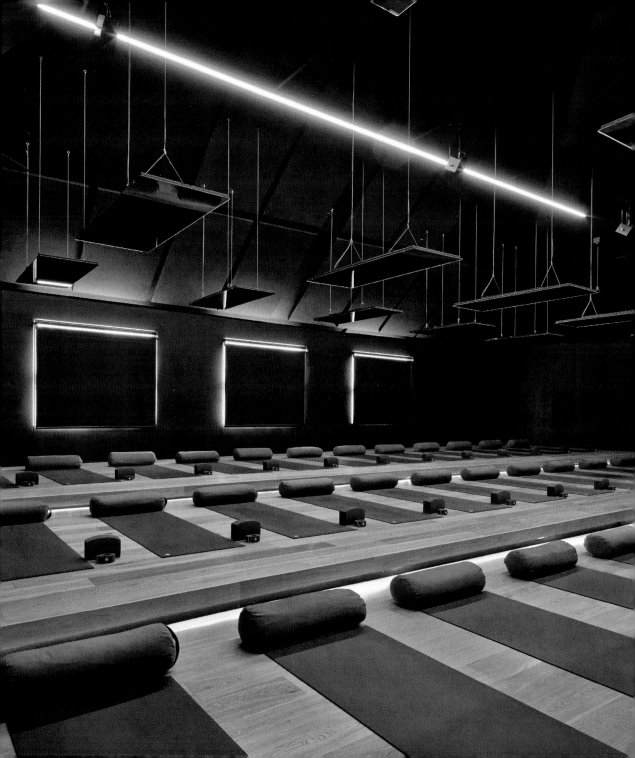

MELBOURNE

RECOMMENDED BY **Jackie Alexander**

Australia is often cited as the West's latecomer to yoga. It wasn't until the mid-1950s, when Chinese-born Westerner Michael Volin came ashore as a refugee from Maoist crackdowns, that Sydney got its first yoga studio. A tiny fad grew around Volin, now better known as Swami Karmananda, as he shared the teachings he learned from his time living with Chinese monks and as a disciple of the revered guru Indra Devi. However, it wasn't really until 1967, when fashion model and yogi pioneer Roma Blair strode into Australian living rooms on *The Don Lane Show* and performed an asana sequence in fishnet tights, that most Australians would consider yoga part of the mainstream.

"I was sort of expecting things to be vastly different here in Melbourne than, say, New York, but the yoga scene here is quite evolved," noted Jackie Alexander. Today, yoga is the number-one preferred method of exercise for most city-dwelling Australians. As with other bustling, cross-cultural hubs like New York City, London, and San Francisco, Melbourne in particular is a city that has come to feature every flavor of yoga, whether you're seeking a slow, mindful, meditative practice, or a body-focused, physically demanding practice. "There's a lot of variety that's really accessible for all types of people. You can pick and choose what works for you. Ashtanga, Sivananda . . . you can find lots of studios that stick to a specific style or lineage, or ones that blend, offering something totally unique."

From the melting pot of lineages that have been brought to Australia's shores, the country's southeast coastal capital is now serving up some truly unique flavors. The city that keeps winning "most livable city" polls also has a famous emphasis on architecture and design. This can be seen at the Crown Casino's massive outdoor fire show, the Recital Centre's facade traced in giant blocks of white neon, or the flamboyantly colored bathing boxes on Brighton Beach. The city's yoga scene is no exception, boasting studios that

OPPOSITE:
Melbourne's
uniquely designed
sound bath studio
by Humming
Puppy has been
described as
"returning to
the womb."

35

place an emphasis on unique design, and the effect this environment can have on a student's physical practice. Studios of note include Simhanada shala and its wild piles of boulders, set to resemble a giant zen garden, or the cheerful flowers and bright walls of Happy Melon, a studio that's more of a house devoted to fitness than a one-room shala.

However, one of the most notable yoga studios to come out of Australia's blend of international influence and unique design is Humming Puppy. Its flagship shala rests in an unassuming building in Melbourne's Prahran neighborhood, a hotspot of hip cafés, specialty boutiques, and vinyl devotees (audiophiles should be sure to visit Greville Records while in the neighborhood). Visitors can walk directly from the heart of this bright, buzzing shopping district into a world of darkness and calm. "We wanted people to feel held from the moment they walked in," Jackie said. This is accomplished by inviting visitors into a space with black walls, underlit lights, no products for sale, and no mirrors up against the wall. With these deliberate design departures from the typical whitewashed, mirror-lined city yoga studio, Humming Puppy produces some of the most blissed-out people you might find in any metropolis. This is largely thanks to the room itself, which, newcomers will note, is humming. "During practice, we inject two frequencies into the room," Jackie explained. "One is 40 hz, the frequency of gamma brain waves—the same waves the brain produces during deep sleep and meditation—and the other is 7.83 hz, which is the frequency of the earth." This "hum" is then set to play in the studio at a rate of 12 bpm—the approximate rate of an ocean wave, or the breathing cycle of a human at rest. The resulting effect on students is overwhelming. "People describe it as a warm hug," Jackie reflected. "I've also heard it compared to returning to the womb or a rolling 'om.'" Both the acoustics of the studio and the "song" itself were designed and perfected by the eminent sound group Arup. Putting the whole design together, from build to acoustics to lights, is no easy feat, but remains an adventurous journey Melbourne has welcomed. "The first time we put on the hum in the room, after going through this huge, stressful, yearlong building process, brought tears to my eyes," Jackie added. "It's like a heartbeat springing to life. It is magic."

Refreshed visitors who leave Humming Puppy looking for more to explore in the coastal capital might find themselves wandering to the Royal Botanic Gardens, a 240-acre complex of fresh greenery, global flora, and tranquil lakes, right in the city center. Water-lovers can head to the coast's famous beaches, some of which may have you doing a double take on your itinerary to ensure you aren't on a tropical island. Walk the long pier over Sorrento Front's cyan waters, cast a line into the smooth, waist-high waves of Half Moon Bay, or catch the horses running on sunny Mordialloc Beach. Just steps away from Port Phillip, Melbourne's poshest neighborhood, sits iconic Brighton Beach, featuring its eighty-two kaleidoscopically colored "bathing boxes," not to mention numerous yoga studios scattered on the shore.

"It's really nice to get back to nature," Jackie remarked of the city. "Melbourne is keen on providing spaces for people to connect to themselves, to each other, and disconnect from the outside world. There is a lot here, for everyone, no matter what you're looking for."

JACKIE ALEXANDER first came to yoga to regain strength and flexibility after a knee injury. She soon became hooked, practicing twice a week with her teacher and developing a daily home practice. In 2013 she left her job managing dental practices and undertook teacher training with the hope to open a studio. Over a cheesy Valentine's Day dinner in 2014 with her partner, Chris, Humming Puppy was conceived. Doors to their first studio in Prahran, Melbourne, opened less than one year later. Humming Puppy also operates studios in Sydney and New York City. When teaching, Jackie favors a breath-centered practice that challenges both the body and the mind to achieve inner awareness.

If You Go

▶ **Getting There**: Melbourne International Airport is served by Delta (800-221-1212; delta.com) and American Airlines (800-433-7300; aa.com).

▶ **Best Time to Visit**: Many people consider spring and fall the best seasons, as they feature moderate temperatures and tourist crowds, plus lower airfare rates. In the summer months (North America's winter months) of December to February, Melbourne is quite busy and very hot.

▶ **Accommodations**: A list of luxe hotels and charming boutique inns is available at visitmelbourne.com.

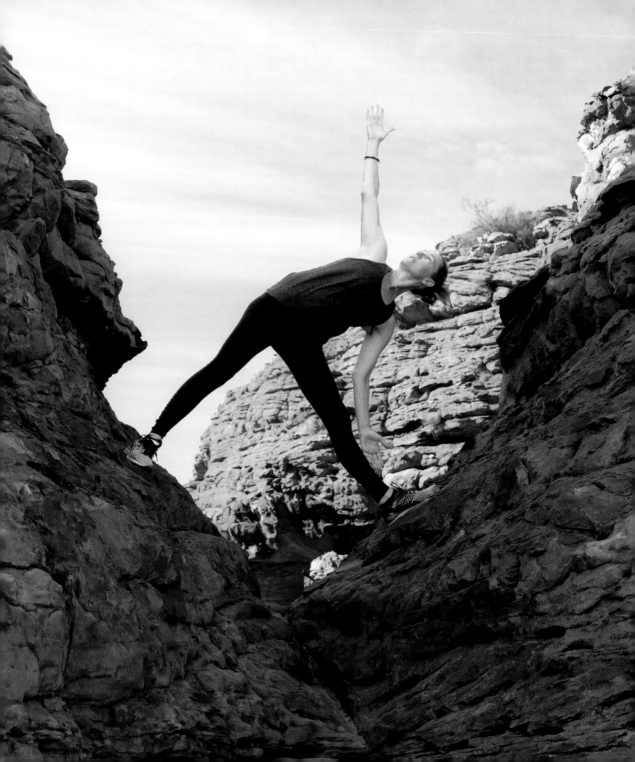

ULURU-KATA TJUTA NATIONAL PARK

RECOMMENDED BY **Denby Sheather**

If you were reared off the island, your list of Australian icons is likely to be populated by kangaroos, koalas, the Sydney Opera House, and, if you're old enough, Crocodile Dundee. But if you're a native Aussie, you're more likely to identify with the massive sandstone edifice of Uluru, sometimes called Ayers Rock. Uluru rests in the southern section of Australia's northern territory, near the continent's geographic center. Reaching a maximum height of 1,143 feet with a circumference of almost six miles, it stands in jarring contrast to the flat and unforgiving environs of Australia's outback; it's now contained within 310,000-acre Uluru-Kata Tjuta National Park. Archaeological research suggests human habitation in the vicinity of Uluru for over ten thousand years; the Anangu believe that their people have been here much longer. According to *Tjukurpa* (the Anangu creation story), nothing existed before the Anangu's ancestors traveled this land. They formed the trees, the rocks, the waterholes, and these features are now proof that these acts of creation took place. Beyond its hulking size and spiritual importance, Uluru also drew both humans and other animals to the springs and waterholes secreted in its sandstone reaches. Kata Tjuta, a group of thirty-six domed rock formations roughly fifteen miles west of Uluru, also has great significance for the Anangu. It's considered the center of knowledge.

It's hard to put into words the spirituality of Uluru and the connections that have existed between it and the people who have inhabited the land for thousands of years. There is an instinctive link that the Anangu (the Aboriginal people of the area) share with their land, the stories of creation and cultural learning as well as significant sites. "To the Anangu, Uluru is everything," Denby Sheather began. "It's the great mother, the protector, the source of life. Uluru is the spiritual heart of Australia. It's also one of the world's

OPPOSITE:
The distinctive
red rocks of
Uluru have had
great spiritual
significance for
the Anangu
for generations.

great energy vortexes and the solar plexus chakra of the planet. When you visit, you feel that energy alongside the wisdom of the Anangu ancestors that have been here for so long. Being at Uluru activates one's instincts and primal memories. Even skeptics feel 'something' indescribable. Uluru is a magical place, and it meets you at the level of consciousness that you are at."

Though she's an Aussie native and a longtime shamanic healer, it was only in recent years that Denby ventured to Uluru. "Back in 2015, the Dalai Lama visited Uluru [in part to advocate for greater protection of Anangu culture]," Denby recalled. "His visit happened to fall around my birthday, so I made the trip north. One morning I hired a car and went to the rock. Walking about, I suddenly felt overwhelmed with its beauty and the healing frequencies. I had an epiphany and was 'told' that I needed to share this place with people so they could gain a deeper experience of the planet and themselves. An elder spirit literally spoke to my heart and gave me permission to bring people here. I had no idea how to bring this about, of course, but I happened to meet a friend of a friend who was an events manager at Ayers Rock Resort [which operates several hotel properties near Uluru] at the exact same time. The manager was keen to bring a wellness retreat to the resort, as it's such a healing place. Everything started flowing and falling into place without any effort, and the retreat, which is called Desert Dreaming, came intuitively." The retreat has now been held five times and is the first wellness retreat to be endorsed by Ayers Rock Resort.

Desert Dreaming is carefully orchestrated. "I like to layer meanings," Denby continued. "I always plan retreats during those weeks when there's a full moon and take other astrological information into consideration as well. The structure of the retreat is more like an intimate story that builds and unfolds over the course of the week. It starts with a Welcome to Country ceremony (known as Inma). If it's possible, we'll have an elder from the Anangu present to help ground our intentions and put us in touch with the land. We'll do a lot conscious walking over the next few days; as you're walking the land, you're walking out your story. If possible, I like to begin at Kata Tjuta and the sacred Valley of the Winds, where we walk with a guide to learn about the spirit guides and power animals that call the valley home. It's a spooky place—in a good way—and you can definitely feel that you're being watched."

A highlight of the retreat is the opportunity to walk all the way around Uluru. "It's a four- to five-hour walk," Denby described, "and we're very careful to respect Anangu customs about not taking photographs where instructed and not going onto the rock itself. We'll stop at various sacred sites around Uluru. Some spots are only for women and some are only for men. The Mutitjulu Waterhole—a women's spot—is one of the most profound on the walk. Even in drought time, there's water present. If you visit Uluru with a pure and open heart, you will receive insights. I've felt hugs and heard voices there, even though no one was around."

At the end of the day, guests retire to the five-star Sails in the Desert Hotel, marked by its soaring white sails and Anangu-inspired decor. (The Mulgara Gallery in the hotel features indigenous artwork, including Anangu dot-paintings.) "We're quite active during the day," Denby shares, "so it's nice to come back to a really comfortable room." Guests are encouraged to indulge in one of the on-premises Red Ochre Spa's treatments as part of their retreat package and, after a lovely dinner, may be treated to a tarot card reading under a full moon.

Of course, each morning begins with a yoga practice. Denby's signature style is called mana yoga. "It has the potential to transform chronic ailments and alleviate the experience of disease in body, mind, and spirit, leaving you feeling physically and mentally grounded, emotionally clear and brave-hearted," she explained. "It's aligned with traditional Chinese medicine and the seasons. As you stretch your organs, you'll also stretch your mind-sets and beliefs so you can be more receptive to the healing powers of Uluru."

Stretching your body and mind as the light of the sunrise plays on Uluru's sandstone walls is certain to be an experience that will stay with you long after you've departed from "down under."

DENBY SHEARER is renowned for her insightful and natural affinity with teaching and her pioneering approach to yoga, health, and healing. Her passion for conscious collaboration led Denby to initiate the Japanese Yoga Teachers Association in Sydney in 2007 and co-found the ocean conservation charity Living Ocean Yoga in 2013. She also founded the innovative practice she calls "mana yoga," a unique flow that reflects her own journey with yoga, energetics, and motherhood. Her latest initiative is Yoga Spirit Journeys, a bespoke, eco-luxe retreat series that seeks to connect people with different cultures through the practices of yoga, meditation, charity, and ceremony. Denby has diplomas in Japanese (Ki) yoga and hatha yoga, Swedish massage, kinergetics, Bowen therapy, and energetic healing. She has trained in mind-body counseling, Theta healing, animal husbandry and healing, shamanic earth-centered practices, soul-retrieval healing, crystal alchemy, aromatherapy, ceremonial work, and meditation. Learn more about her work at denbysheather.com.

If You Go

▶ **Getting There**: Visitors can fly into Yulara from Sydney on Jetstar (866-397-8170; jetstar.com) and through Alice Springs on Qantas (800-227-4500; qantas.com.au).

▶ **Best Time to Visit**: The weather in the Northern Territory is cooler in the Aussie fall and winter, between May and September.

▶ **Accommodations**: Ayers Rock Resort (+61 889577001; ayersrockresort.com.au) is home to a number of lodging options, including Sails in the Desert, the site of Desert Dreaming. For more information about Desert Dreaming, contact Yoga Spirit Journeys (+61 413747644); yogaspiritjourneys.com.

ST. ANTON AM ARLBERG

RECOMMENDED BY **Iris Kaufmann**

The alpine villages of Austria's Tyrol Mountains are known for attracting more skiers than yogis, especially in St. Anton. The tidy village of just 2,500 inhabitants is a perfect picture of rustic Tyrolean charm, especially in the dark of winter. Skiers rejoice in the nearly 200 miles (300 km) of marked ski runs and eighty-eight lift areas. But the magic of crisp Alps air and white clouds twirling amid evergreen boughs persists far beyond winter. "In the summer, it's a much different experience," began Kaufmann. "It's extremely peaceful, and the town is literally surrounded by beautiful green mountains and flowers and the cleanest air you've ever breathed."

The Mountain Yoga Festival has only been running since 2015 but already has had to cap its ticket sales to 250. Yogis used to the thousand-yard crowds at the yoga festivals of South Asia will find themselves taken aback by the intimacy of this retreat. "We try to keep it small because that's what makes it so special," continued Iris. "We don't have hundreds of people in the classes, there's more room for teachers to see you and give you feedback, and for people to actually connect with each other."

Aside from the chance to connect with yogis from across the globe and learn from some of Europe's best teachers in an intimate setting, the Mountain Yoga Festival is a rare opportunity to commune with some of Europe's most treasured mountainscapes. "From the beginning, we had a focus on not just yoga, but nature as well," noted Iris. "We're surrounded by mountains up here, and we are mountain people. Our meditation is hiking and walking."

The four-day festival works with and through the flowery meadows, airy mountaintops, misty forest glades, and rocky slopes surrounding St. Anton. Each day begins with a morning meditation and a hearty vegetarian communal breakfast, followed by a ride in the

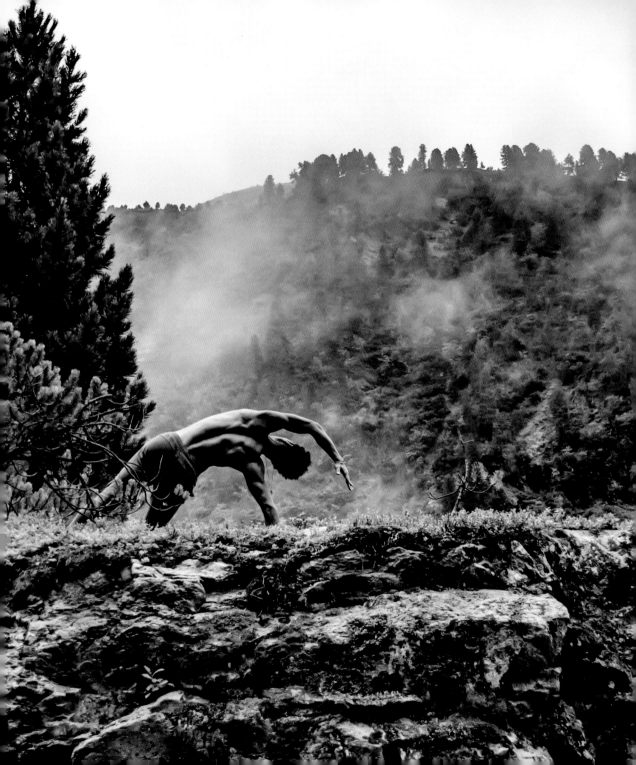

chairlift to the mountain's upper limits," explained Iris, "and there's a ski hut up there we have use of all summer. It has a sloped roof made of wood, very traditional. Of course, if the weather is good, we roll the mats open outside and practice right in the meadow with the grass, flowers, and clouds that usually come around and pass through us."

After a communal lunch, a variety of afternoon workshops are available for guests. "Maybe there's a talk on balancing the chakras, or someone giving a lecture about nutrition or hiking," Iris continued. "We talk about the benefits you can get from the trees and the air and the soft ground. One of the big things we have at almost any time of day at the festival is "yoga hikes," led by local guides. You can start in the morning and hike to a specific place, like a secluded mountain hut, and along the way you'll stop and listen to the water trickling down the mountain, or observe the animals, or feel the leaves of a pine tree. Then, when you arrive at the hut, you can grab a cup of tea and sit. We like to take people through an exercise, asking them 'Why is the air different up here?' 'What does it do with your eyes?' or 'How do you feel in this moment?' We also offer a sunrise hike if the weather is willing, starting at 4:30 A.M. We hike up the mountain, and then we do yoga with the sunrise. It's quite cold, but it's one of those moments that completely takes you over. It is so quiet in the morning, maybe nothing but the bells of the sheep next to you."

One of the perks of being part of a retreat in a town so small is the opportunity for meaningful connection. "The festival takes up the whole village," reflected Iris. "Everything is within walking distance. Maybe you're staying in a hotel or a B&B, but everyone you see in your accommodation, or at a restaurant, or on the street walking about, is, by day 4, someone you probably know.

"There were already a few yogis here practicing before we set up the festival, but yoga is not really part of the traditional history here. Day 1 of the first festival was interesting. The locals were kind of curious. Some of them were saying, 'Oh no, will they run barefoot through the village with dreadlocks?' They had this kind of negative stereotype of what yogis are. Obviously it was totally different. The participants showed up and they were moms, managers, students, normal people from all over the world. Then some locals started joining the festival, opening up their hotels or restaurants with things that cater to the crowd. It's something the entire town now looks forward to after ski season."

Can a yoga festival bring even greater tranquility to a mountain town? Iris shared a story that suggests it can be so. "On our third year, there was an older local man named

OPPOSITE:
A skier's paradise
in the winter,
St. Anton bursts
with greenery
in the summer,
allowing yogis
to practice
in the clouds.

Manfred who was with us the whole four days. He's been practicing yoga in St. Anton for a very long time. After the closing ceremony, he came up to me and said, 'With this festival, you are giving a peacefulness back to the locals, to the village, that's really needed. St. Anton is very loud and busy in winter, and with this festival it's like a cover where people can recharge. It's so much positive energy.'"

IRIS KAUFMANN was born and raised in the Austrian Alps. She's been working in the marketing and tourism field for the last twenty years. She first connected to yoga while living in Sydney in 2008 and has been practicing wherever she can roll out the mat ever since. Yoga is part of her life, like brushing one's teeth in the morning. Although she completed a teacher training in India, to deepen her yoga experience, she is currently not teaching private classes. Instead, she loves to combine her marketing and yoga experience by organizing the Mountain Yoga Festival St. Anton for the world to enjoy a new perspective on yoga.

If You Go

▶ **Getting There**: Innsbruck Airport is the closest, and served by Lufthansa (800-645-3880; lufthansa.com) and British Airways (800-247-9297; britishairways.com). From there, a car or train can take you directly into St. Anton. Zurich Airport, although farther away, is served by more international carriers, although your train ride will be a little longer.
▶ **Best Time to Visit**: The Mountain Yoga Festival in St. Anton takes place in late summer, typically August or early September. Winter is also a spectacular time to visit, if you are ready for snow.
▶ **Accommodations**: The town has about seventy-five accommodation options, from five-star hotels such as Hotel Tannenhof (+43 544630311; hoteltannenhof.net) to earthy farm-stays such as Hotel Garni Bergwelt (+43 54462995; bergwelttirol.com). St. Anton am Arlberg Tourism Office (+43 544622690; stantonamarlberg.com) lists the region's many lodging options.

PARADISE ISLAND

RECOMMENDED BY **Rukmini Chaitanya**

As a destination for those craving a quintessential tropical paradise vacation, the Bahamas needs hardly any introduction. The nation of many islands just off the east coast of Florida hosts a tidy number of yoga studios to serve vacationers seeking a soft-sanded, palm-shaded environment on which to reflect, meditate, and grow their practice. However, on the aptly named "Paradise Island," just off the coast of New Providence, the Sivananda Ashram Yoga Retreat awaits yogis seeking a more traditionally grounded, service-oriented ashram, ready to help you center on a deeper level of spiritual commitment.

The Sivananda Ashram Yoga Retreat Bahamas is part of the International Yoga Vedanta Centre, which is one of the largest training centers for yoga teachers in the world, having produced nearly fifty thousand graduates since 1969. Founded by Swami Vishnudevananda Saraswati—the twentieth century's famous "flying swami" who introduced yoga to the Beatles in the 1960s, "bombed" India and Pakistan and other conflict areas in the world with flowers and peace pamphlets in 1971, and flew over the Berlin Wall during the Cold War in 1983—the center was built in response to a calling from the Divine. Swami Vishnudevananda was sent from India to the West in 1957 by his teacher, the renowned yoga master, Swami Sivananda, who is considered one of the greatest saints of India in the twentieth century. Swami Vishnudevananda founded the International Sivananda Yoga Vedanta Centre in 1959 with the goal to share the science of yoga and Vedanta with people all over the world.

"There is a rock on the property, in the main ashram temple," Rukmini Chaitanya began, "where Swami Vishnudevananda had a profound vision in 1969. This was before it was an altar—it was just a rock. He was sitting before it, and meditating, and he had an

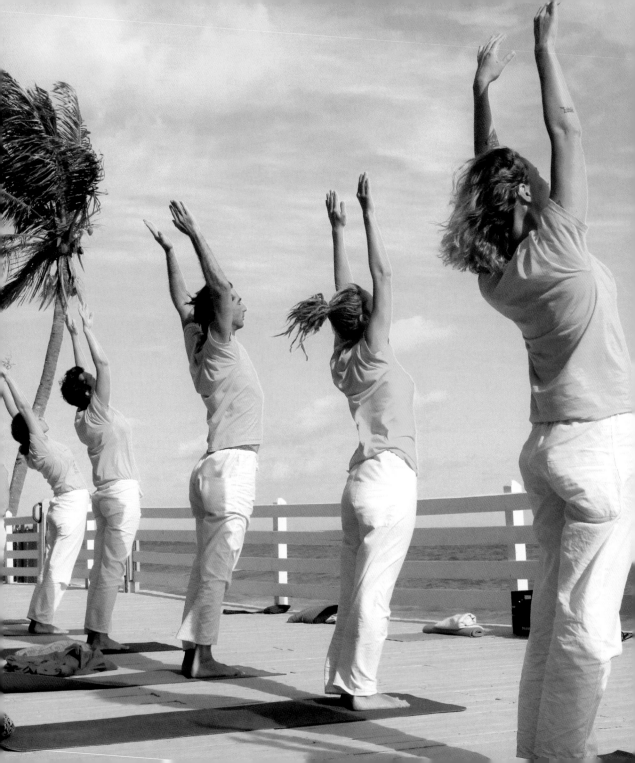

experience that led him to start this mission of bringing yoga all over the world, to bring people together, to break borders, break racial boundaries, break religious and cultural boundaries. He had a vision that humanity must unite if we want to make it to the next century together. This rock is now our main altar and around it is our main temple. It's a very powerful place."

Sivananda is situated between Nassau harbor and the sapphire vastness of the Atlantic, surrounded by pristine white sand beaches, radiant blue waters, and five and a half acres of lush gardens (Judith Hanson Lasater, co-founder of the West's first yoga magazine, *Yoga Journal*, took her honeymoon there in the early 1970s). "The first time I came, I intended to stay for two weeks. I ended up staying for seven," reflected Rukmini Chaitanya. "I knew then I wanted to join the organization. It took some time before I could free myself of my academic career—I started doing yoga to manage stress during my PhD program—but eventually I became full-time at the organization and stayed primarily based in the Bahamas. That was twenty years ago. I could not be happier."

From private, spacious rooms that overlook the ocean to tent huts tucked into the jungle, the center houses students, karma yogis, and guests coming for one of the ashram's many specialty retreats or workshops (featuring bestselling authors, teachers, and kirtan singers such as Krishna Das and John Perkins).

The ashram's daily offerings begin at six A.M. with morning satsang (guided silent meditation followed by chanting and a lecture). The day continues with asana/pranayama practices for all levels; meals, workshops, and beach time; and it ends with evening satsang, when again everyone gathers for meditation, chanting, and a talk or performance by a guest speaker or artist. "About two days a week, instead of meeting in the satsang hall in the early morning, we do a silent walk on the beach, as well as a sunrise meditation next to the water," said Rukmini Chaitanya. Those who visit as vacationers, as well as those who are volunteers or students, would do well to explore the many treatments in the Wellbeing Center, whose menu includes Ayurvedic consultation, Ayurveda body treatments, therapeutic massage, Thai massage, reflexology, and more.

Any visitor would be remiss if they didn't dangle their toes into the Bahamas' postcard-perfect water. "The beach is what we are most known for," Rukmini Chaitanya continued. "The ocean in this area of the Bahamas is stunningly beautiful. You get all the gradients of the blue color: the turquoise, the deep blue, the light blue, and then, of course, the color of

OPPOSITE:
Paradise Island offers yogis a meditative, lush backdrop for a vigorous and internationally respected training program.

the sky . . . and it's all framed by coconut trees. If you live here, you have this view over your eyes 24/7. You can feel the expansiveness of creation. For many people who come here, the beach is a sacred place. It's not literally a temple, but . . . of course it's a temple." Scuba diving, snorkeling, and boating all invite you to explore the sea.

Visitors looking to connect with the magic of the tropical jungle will appreciate the care that the ashram has fostered with the natural world, leading to a delightful relationship with local Bahamian flora and fauna. "One of my favorite places at the ashram is a small temple we keep in the middle of the forest, called Vana Durga (which literally translates to 'mother of the forest' or 'Divine mother'). We refer to it as the Golden Wood. There is a rope around it. We don't cultivate the garden there; we let it grow wildly, leaving it there for nature and for the nature beings. We have a small temple there for the Divine mother, but we don't allow anyone in there unless it's during a particular ceremony."

Garden visitors will also notice an incredible array of animals, at home in the nourished and wild jungle. "There are so many birds here," Rukmini Chaitanya said. "We make a point to take care of the garden and nature, and so the birds feel very happy to hang around. There are also lizards, geckos . . . and, of course, incredibly beautiful fish," Rukmini Chaitanya said. "We have a dog and a few cats that have adopted us, but mostly we have birds and lizards as our pets."

Guests who find that a week's visit is not enough are welcome to pursue the residential study program, a volunteer program of devoted karma yogis who study, serve, and grow their spiritual selves while making everything happen behind the scenes. "Our slogan here in Paradise is to *expand your horizons*," Rukmini Chaitanya added. "When you look at the ocean, you get this feeling of expansiveness. You look at it, and you see there's no limit, no end. This is what we want you to feel you can do. But truly, what this slogan means for us is to expand your mind, expand your knowledge, come and learn from world-renowned teachers, healers, artists, and spiritual practitioners, from all walks of life, all cultures, nations, and traditions. Our motto, which we inherited from our teachers, Swami Sivananda and Swami Vishnudevananda, is Unity in Diversity—all are welcome, all are Divine, all are one."

RUKMINI CHAITANYA is a senior member of the Sivananda Ashram Yoga Retreat and personal assistant to Swami Swaroopananda, the ashram director. A knowledgeable and experienced teacher and yoga practitioner, she has been teaching yoga classes and offering lectures on Sivananda yoga philosophy for nearly twenty years.

If You Go

▶ **Getting There**: Fly into Nassau International Airport, served by several airlines including Bahamasair (242-702-4140; bahamasair.com) and American Airlines (800-433-7300; aa.com), and then give the ashram a call so it can prepare a boat for you. Take a taxi from the airport to the Elizabeth on Bay Marketplace and Marina in downtown Nassau, and a boat will be waiting to take you to Paradise Island.

▶ **Best Time to Visit**: Many consider the best time to visit the Bahamas to be between mid-December and mid-April. Though temperatures rarely dip below 60 degrees Fahrenheit year-round, hurricanes may be a factor beginning in June, and especially through the fall.

▶ **Accommodations**: The Sivananda Ashram is bookable for a variety of vacation packages and more focused yoga programs at sivanandabahamas.org. Other accommodations on the island can be found with the Bahamas Tourism Board at bahamas.com.

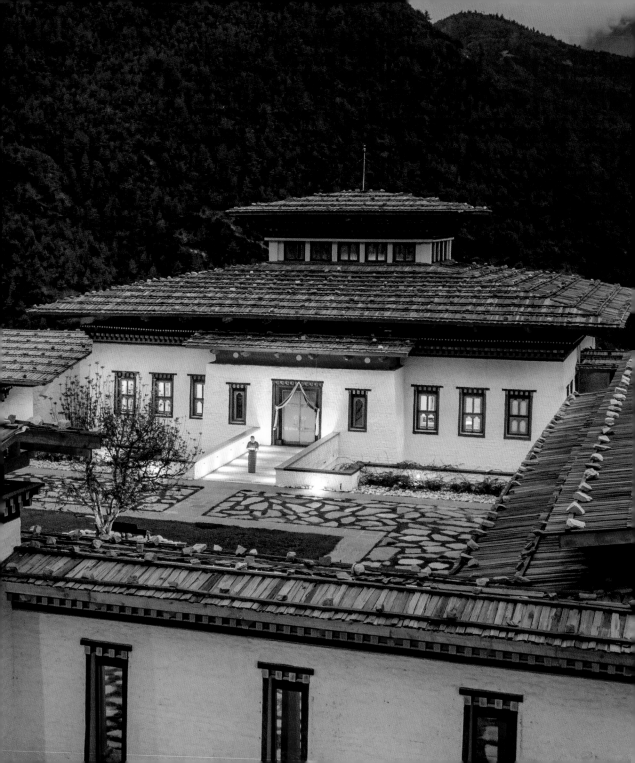

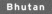

PARO

RECOMMENDED BY **Louk Lennaerts**

"We're in stress at home," Louk Lennarts began. "And we take this stress on holidays, with our itineraries and this feeling of 'We have to see this, and we have to see that . . .' It's as if we're doing a job again, rather than finding a place where we can connect to ourselves. Bhutan really is a place where you can rest. Maybe it's because so many monks have been doing prayers here for hundreds of years. Maybe it's because the country has been isolated. All I know is that people have a different mind-set here. It's slower. The air is like magic. It is famous for its sustainability—they produce a negative CO_2 balance. You can't find this in India, it's too busy. Thailand has famous places for yoga, but none of them are like Bhutan."

All but floating in the clouds between India and Tibet, Bhutan is a country that has kept itself deliberately hidden from the world. Never colonized, the Buddhist kingdom did not even open its doors to foreign entry until 1974. Today, although the visa cap has been increasing, the Tourism Council of Bhutan upholds a strict policy to preserve the country's unique landscape and culture.

"The Bhutanese use happiness, not money, as a major direction of measuring their progress," Louk observed. "Coming here, you can get inspired and see that it's possible to live differently. Globally, mindfulness is becoming something very popular, something that is for everybody. This is a place where you can see mindfulness energy affecting everything. And why shouldn't tourism be the right vehicle to mobilize people to look at their lives a little bit differently?"

The influence of Bhutanese culture is evident from the moment you enter the Bhutan Spirit Sanctuary, an all-inclusive paradise perched in the eastern mountains, surrounded by evergreen trees and golden grasses. "We call it the transformation room," described

OPPOSITE:
The world's
happiest country
welcomes new
and seasoned
yogis alike.

Louk. "To enter the Sanctuary, you walk into a courtyard, cross a small golden bridge to the main building, and enter into a small ritual room, where a traditional Bhutanese ritual is performed. You enter, find a butter lamp, light it, and observe the paintings on the wall that explain the culture of Bhutan. Then, we open the big golden doors, and you look right into the Neyphu valley. People really arrive feeling that something has happened. And yes, something has happened. You are in Bhutan now."

Though not dedicated expressly to yoga, the Sanctuary ends up converting more than a few of its guests to the practice. "A lot of guests don't come because they see we do yoga and meditation," remarked Louk. "But people who do visit will often try. We believe yoga is for every person, and it's not just something for the muscles. It's a way to find inner balance."

The wellness benefits of a Sanctuary stay extend beyond yoga. Guests can attend a session with a traditional Bhutanese medicine doctor to help diagnose and cure any ailments, as well as a variety of herbal body health treatments, from medicine to massage. "Bhutan is famous for its herbs," Louk continued. One favorite treatment involves soaking in a hot stone herbal bath—where large stones, freshly warmed on the fire, are placed in a large tub with you, enriching the water with heat and minerals.

This treatment might be just the ticket after spending a day of high-altitude hiking to visit Bhutan's famed floating Paro Taktsang (aka "Tiger's Nest,"), a grand, white and red monastery that appears to be hanging directly off the side of sheer granite cliffs. Closer to the Sanctuary, a smaller, active monastery welcomes curious visitors. "You can walk over," explained Louk. "There's a head monk who talks to visitors, and a Buddhism school for young students. The guests can chat with the monks and the monks with the guests. The valley is quite exclusive, so the monks still enjoy receiving guests." If they prefer, guests can also enjoy the view of the monastery from the Sanctuary itself. "From each room, the indoor heated pool, the restaurant, and every other place in the Sanctuary, you can see the mountains on one side, and the valley on the other, and the monastery across from us," Louk added. "I love to open the curtains in the morning and see the sky on top—the clouds are sometimes floating in the monastery."

"I really think of this place and Bhutan as a whole, as a sanctuary. Not a hotel, or a resort, but a Sanctuary." Louk opined. "This means taking care of people in a different way, in a more familial atmosphere. We don't take your credit card or passport at reception; we know who you are. Everything, all the treatments and services and meals, are included. I don't think people would try new things like yoga and herbal teas if we charged extra for it."

Visitors who are lucky enough to make the trip often laud Bhutan as the real-life Shangri-La, and the country is set on preserving this reputation for generations to come. "In yoga," concluded Louk, "we look for an environment that gives us energy. Bhutan gives that certain energy. Our inner sustainability is fostered by this outer sustainability. I know these can sound like empty words, but once you're here, you will understand."

LOUK LENNAERTS used to work in emerging tourism markets in Eastern Europe. After a journey founding fusion Maia resorts, Danang, and others in Vietnam in the early 2000s, he traveled to Bhutan with the plan to explore and rest. It was there that the Bhutanese Rinpoche, His Eminence Gyalwa Dokhampa, gave Louk a copy of his book titled *The Restful Mind*, and Louk found the way to integrate his own inner journey for a restful mind with the project to build a true Sanctuary. The result was the founding of a resort where guests can feel like a part of Bhutan and not a mere tourist, inspired by the Bhutanese culture, the compassionate people of Bhutan, and the Buddhist path to enlightenment.

If You Go

▶ **Getting There**: Most flights connect to Bhutan through Delhi, Bangkok, or Kathmandu. Bhutan Spirit Sanctuary is a twenty-minute shuttle drive from Paro Airport, Bhutan's only international airport, served by Drukair (+65 63389909; drukair.com) and Bhutan Airlines (+975 77106011; bhutanairlines.bt).

▶ **Best Time to Visit**: October to December is considered the ideal time to visit Bhutan. January and February are colder. In late spring the famous rhododendrons bloom, flooding the valleys with color, followed by a humid summer and the monsoon season from June through September.

▶ **Accommodations**: Bhutan Spirit Sanctuary is bookable at bhutanspiritsanctuary.com, and the Bhutan Tourism Board offers additional hotels at tourism.gov.bt.

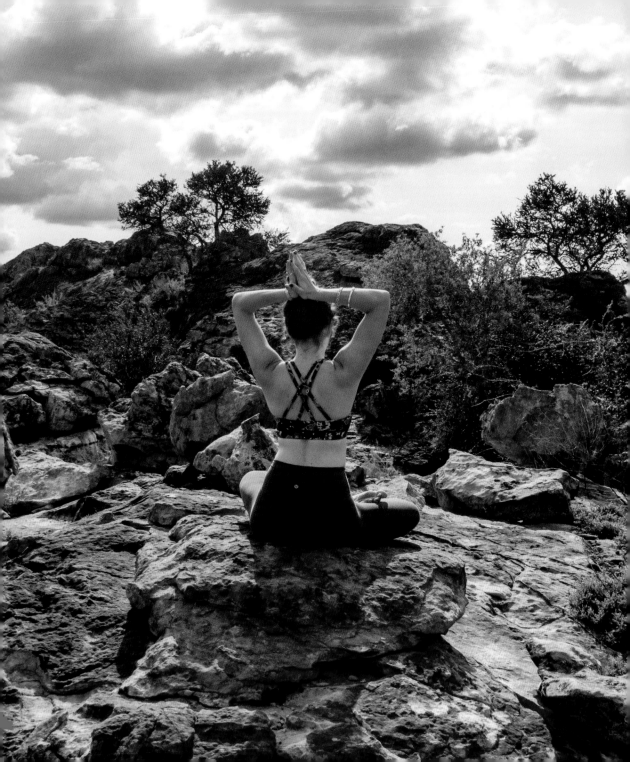

WELGEVONDEN GAME RESERVE / TULI RESERVE

RECOMMENDED BY **Lauren Lalita Duker**

For some, yoga is about connecting with the life source, the larger rhythms of Mother Earth. In this respect, there may be no better place to practice than on safari in the African bushveldt, among some of the world's most charismatic animals.

"We find that yoga is one of the most beautiful and natural things to bring to a safari," Lauren Duker began. "The mindful aspect of practice allows you to slow down and savor the moment. On many safaris, it's all about seeing the 'Big Five' and checking the next animal off the list. On a yoga safari, it's much more about connecting with nature and oneself. The day is bookmarked by sunrise and sunset, the times when the bushveldt comes to life. In that border between night and day, there are moments of illumination. It's a place of profound connection.

"The physical aspects of yoga are also an excellent complement to a safari. You need exercise, but you can't head out for a walk or a jog at most lodges, as there are wild animals around. Having a chance to practice yoga gets the body moving. It's one of the keys to feeling good."

Lauren and her cohorts at Euphoria Retreats have assembled several yoga safaris over the years. The itinerary that's closet to her heart splits time between South Africa and Botswana. "We start at Sediba Lodge, a luxurious property that sits between tree canopies in the Welgevonden Game Reserve," Lauren continued. "It's a stunning location, with wonderful amenities like hot tubs overlooking the bushveldt in each suite. But it's a warm and welcoming luxury that makes you feel at home, not hoity-toity. As the name implies, this reserve is home to Africa's 'Big Five' animals—lions, leopards, Cape buffalo, black rhino, and elephants. This is a wilderness area, so you're not guaranteed to see them all, although our yoga retreat guests have, including some rare

OPPOSITE:
Yogis visiting Tuli
and Welgevonden
Game Reserve
mix practice
with safari-style
game viewing.

leopard sightings. The rangers in the park are very experienced and knowledgeable; it seems like magic how they know where and when to go to find animals. They are able to get us incredibly close. Sometimes when you come upon animals it's startling. You don't always know what's happening, but the guides do.

"After several days at Sediba, we cross into Botswana. It's an unconventional border passage, as we take a tram that's pulled across the Limpopo River. We might spy hippos below as we cross! Our home in Botswana is the Tuli Safari Lodge in the Tuli Reserve, which is renowned for some of the largest elephant herds in Africa. On our last trip there, the group encountered a bull elephant right on one of the roads leading to the bushveldt. He was so large and intimidating, it was almost otherworldly." It's not unheard of for guests to come upon herds of up to forty elephants, including babies. You're also sure to come upon most of the other animals that call the bushveldt home—giraffes, warthogs, zebras, antelopes, wildebeest, baboons, hyenas, and ostriches. Birders will find more than three hundred species. "The lodge rests among rugged sandstone formations and Baobab trees, the flora you probably associate with the bushveldt," Lauren said. "It's really interwoven with the surrounding environment; sometimes animals will come walking through. It has a pool, gardens and walking trails, and beautifully appointed tent cabins, but to me, its most defining feature is the star deck. When you sit out there in the evening, the canopy above is unbelievable."

Safari drives or bush walks—sometimes a combination of the two—are held during the low light times, daybreak and late afternoon. "During the morning drive, we practice mindfulness," Lauren described. "On bush drives there can be a lot of talking as we learn about the wildlife. We also take a few moments to stay silent, breathe, listen to the bush, and connect to the rhythms of nature. As the heat rises, the animals seek shelter. We do the same. Back at the lodge, we have a lazy brunch, and then there's time to rest or take a swim. Mid-afternoon, we'll have a yoga session with one of our guest instructors. Our teacher for 2021 is Nina Butler, from South Africa. Her practice is vinyasa-oriented. The yoga style that's practiced on a given trip will depend on the instructor. Though styles may vary, all of our teachers are world-class and experienced teaching to people of all levels, from beginners to other teachers. Once the yoga session is done, we set out for our sunset safari. As radiant colors light up the horizon, we'll have a drink—a "sundowner"—to toast the day, the people, and place. It's a beautiful, mindful savoring of the experience as we stop and take it all in. We typically dine al fresco, under the brilliant night sky, to maintain that connection to nature. All the cuisine is exquisite; guests may not be expecting how good it's going to be." (Meat is served at some meals, though the chefs at Sediba and Tuli can accommodate any dietary preferences.)

"Some yoga retreats can be a bit austere, and intentionally so," Lauren added. "Their intent may be to help attendees detox. The trips Euphoria Retreats creates are meant to be yoga holidays. We have yoga and meditation yes, but also fine dining, good wines, and luxe surroundings. We like to say that on one of our retreats, yoga is optional, but good food and wine is not."

The animals of the bushveldt are the prime attraction of a yoga safari. But there's also an opportunity to glimpse the region's rich human history at Mapungubwe, where the remains of a flourishing Iron Age kingdom dating back to 900 CE can be toured.

"Our safari experiences have given us so many great memories," Lauren shared. "What I love most are those sunsets as the jeep stops and we lift our sundowners. The sky is ablaze with orange, red, and pink. Watching the sun sink, we're connected both to nature and to each other."

LAUREN LALITA DUKER is a yoga instructor who unites new science and ancient tradition as she weaves anatomical movement with ancient practices. Lauren's teaching is designed to open you to the joys of each moment. Her voice, in guided meditation or song, will help move you into deeper states of awareness. Off the mat, Lauren manages client relations and sales for Euphoria Retreats from her home in Northern California.

If You Go

▶ **Getting There**: Trips stage in Johannesburg, South Africa, which is served by many major carriers. Guests will generally overnight at the Intercontinental Hotel (ihg.com) at the Tambo airport before beginning their adventure the following day.

▶ **Best Time to Visit**: This trip is generally offered in April.

▶ **Accommodations**: Euphoria Retreats (970-924-0253; euphoriaretreats.com) coordinates all aspects of the yoga safari, including lodging at Sediba and Tuli Lodges, meals, guides, and transportation between venues.

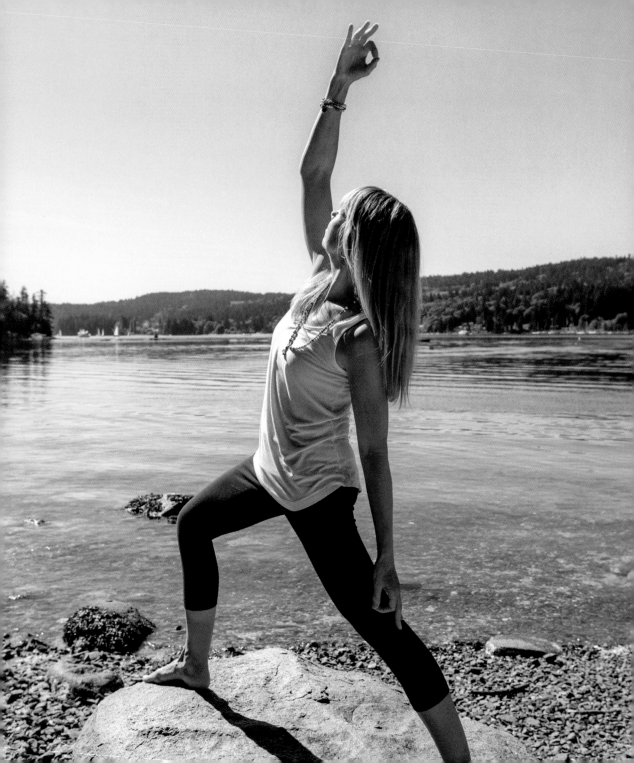

SALT SPRING ISLAND

RECOMMENDED BY **Sharada Filkow**

Tucked between mainland British Columbia and Vancouver Island, Salt Spring Island is as idyllic a coastal retreat as one can imagine. It's no wonder that it's become the site of a renowned yoga retreat. However, as Sharada Filkow recalled, the choice of Salt Spring was not immediate.

"I first met our teacher, Baba Hari Dass—affectionately known as Babaji, 'respected father'—in 1971," Sharada Filkow began. "By the mid-seventies, a few others and I formed Dharma Sara Satsang Society in Vancouver to practice classical ashtanga yoga, long before it was so popular. We started holding summer retreats, and we'd attract three hundred or four hundred people. Our core group of thirty or forty decided that we should establish a permanent home. Portions of the group would go on scouting expeditions around British Columbia and Alberta. They'd come back saying, 'We found the greatest place!' But others in our group would respond, 'We don't want to live on a mountain!' It wasn't easy to get everyone on board. But when someone suggested Salt Spring Island, we all agreed. It felt like a place where people could experience healthy, peaceful living. We bought the land in 1981 and began renovations on the main building, a farmhouse that had been built in 1911. As soon as it was habitable, we began running programs."

Salt Spring Island is the most populous of British Columbia's Gulf Islands, which are a northern extension of Washington State's San Juan Islands. Nestled in the Strait of Georgia, Salt Spring offers picturesque ocean views and hospitable harbors that are reminiscent of northern New England. During summer months, the island attracts many visitors, eager to kayak, stand-up paddleboard, hike, and browse the island's art galleries. Many visitors will venture to the island via ferry, and it's common to see orcas (killer whales) as you sail to and fro.

OPPOSITE:
Salt Spring
Island is
among the
most beautiful
of BC's
Gulf Islands
and is home
to Salt Spring
Centre.

Though Salt Spring Island has abundant diversions, many retreat attendees choose to stay on the premises of Salt Spring Centre. "The property is just under seventy acres," Sharada continued. "There are big conifers sprinkled among the meadows and farmlands and a seasonal stream that's followed by a trail. The property is also a short walk to a lake. We have a big organic garden on the property, and that's helped us build a reputation for our food. In fact, we've published two vegetarian cookbooks."

In the early days, Salt Spring Centre sponsored women's weekends. These morphed into yoga getaways. "There are a number of ways that people come to experience the Centre, and our monthly yoga getaways are one of the most popular," Sharada said. "Salt Spring is a place where you can come, have a break, focus on treatment, and relax. It's amazing what can happen in the span of a weekend. By Saturday evening, guests are relaxing. By Sunday, they're transformed. Many guests come back every year." In addition to weekend retreats, Salt Spring Centre holds summer teacher training sessions, ten-week karma yoga programs, and an annual yoga retreat the first weekend in August. "The annual retreats have lots of options for classes and a tremendous community feeling," Sharada added. "Families are welcome, and we have a fabulous program for kids while their parents are in classes." It should be noted that Salt Spring Centre is an intentional, working community with a strong focus on karma yoga (the yoga of action, or selfless service.)

As mentioned above, the teaching program at Salt Spring is focused on classical ashtanga yoga, first set forth by the sage Patanjali in his "Yoga Sutras," nearly two thousand years ago. Ashtanga translates as "eight-limbed" and speaks to the eight facets of the practice:

- Yamas (Restraints), including nonviolence, truthfulness, non-stealing, continence, and non-hoarding
- Niyamas (Observances), including purity, contentment, austerity, scriptural study, surrender to God
- Asana (Posture), the meditation postures that promote concentration and a strong, flexible body
- Pranayama (Breath Control), to expand life-support energy
- Pratyahara (Withdrawing the Mind from Sense Perception), to liberate the senses from the objects that attract them
- Dharana (Concentration), to train the mind to dwell only on a chosen object
- Dhyana (Meditation), the channeling of the mind to one point
- Samadhi (Super Consciousness), for complete absorption in one object

Sharada has many happy memories of Babaji, a silent monk who was her teacher for fifty years. "He'd come here twice a year in the early days, later once a year. [Babaji was based in California, at Mount Madonna Center, near Santa Cruz.] When he was able to visit, we'd do a lot of work parties as a community. There are many rock walls here that we built; such rock walls and temples were common in northern India where he came from. He liked projects that everyone could take part in. The kinds of projects that he initiated still happen.

"I often think of a quote from Babaji, who wrote:

"Work honestly. Meditate every day. Meet people without fear. Play.

"We used to think, *OK, work honestly*—we do that. We're working on the meditation. We have fun, so we play. We thought we were meeting people without fear, but maybe we weren't. To do so, you need to remain present, to be there completely. It's still an ongoing practice."

SHARADA FILKOW is a karma yogi, a teacher of yoga philosophy and nonviolent communication, and a mentor. An elder in Dharma Sara Satsang Society, she's been at Salt Spring Centre since 1983.

If You Go

► **Getting There**: Guests can travel to Salt Spring Island by ferry from Vancouver or Victoria (bcferries.com) or via seaplane (harbourair.com) from Vancouver and several sites on Vancouver Island. Victoria is served by several carriers, including Air Canada (888-247-2262; aircanada.com) and Horizon Air (800-252-7522; alaskaair.com).

► **Best Time to Visit**: Salt Spring Centre (250-537-2326; saltspringcentre.com) offers retreats every month of the year. The Centre's Annual Community Yoga Retreat is generally held in early August. Yoga teacher training is offered over two sessions in the summer months.

► **Accommodations**: Yoga Getaways include lodging in the Centre's farmhouse, classes, and fine vegetarian cuisine.

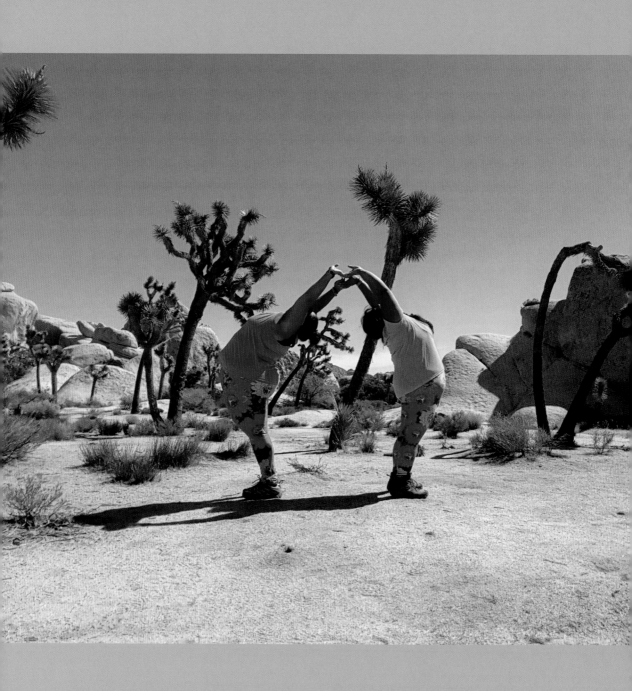

JOSHUA TREE

RECOMMENDED BY **Jessica Rihal**

The alien desert realm of monolithic boulders and tufted, Seussian trees known as Joshua Tree National Park sits 111 miles east of Los Angeles. The trees and park earned their name from Mormon settlers who believed the tree branches they saw while crossing the desert were the arms of Joshua, beckoning them toward the Promised Land. Today, although named for its distinctive vegetation, Joshua Tree is better known as the "rock climber's Mecca," due to its massive, hallucinatory rock formations that span the length of city blocks. However, one doesn't need to be a rock climber to enjoy this majestic marriage zone of the Colorado and Mojave Desert. It's attracted hippies, wanderlusters, and spiritual seekers for generations.

Some yogis are drawn here for the Institute of Mentalphysics Joshua Tree Retreat Center, "the physical manifestation of the desert's spirituality," which offers a wide variety of workshops from leaders in mindfulness, meditation, and a variety of yoga styles. Others come here as a part of private, organized retreats such as "Desert Reset," which offers hypnotherapy-based, vegan yoga for those wishing to harness the energy of the desert to transform their lives. The town of Joshua Tree, located just outside the park boundary, has its own yoga studios, such as Instant Karma. Numerous LA–based studios offer day or weeklong retreats for their city-dwelling clients to plug into this naked energy. Deep Yoga, a San Diego–based studio, offers "Yoga Rocks!" a special retreat that combines the unapparelled rock-climbing routes with asana practices.

However, perhaps one of Joshua Tree's most notable perks is that you need not arrive with an an organized retreat group—merely some camping equipment and an open mind.

"Being in scenic places was a love I developed later in life," began Jessica Rihal. "My mom didn't want us hurting ourselves, so we didn't go camping when I was young. I was

OPPOSITE:
Yogis greet the
dawn camping
among Joshua
Tree's signature
tufted boughs.

quite skeptical the first time I came to Joshua Tree. I'm from Orange County, which is very suburban. At that point in my life, the only time I'd ever been camping was at Newport Dunes—you can hear cars going by and there's a general store, so it's not really 'roughing it.' So, Joshua Tree was the first time I actually went camping. I loved it."

As a national park, Joshua Tree offers a variety of developed, drive-up campsites that provide all basic amenities—restrooms, fire-rings, and picnic tables—and can be reserved in advance. Those seeking a more intimate adventure with the desert can obtain backpacker's permits and hike for miles across the 800,000-acre park. In summer, America's camping season, visitors may find it difficult to secure a camping spot, despite the threat of daytime temperatures that soar above 100 degrees Fahrenheit. However, autumn and winter campers, especially around the holidays, may find themselves pleasantly surprised to have this otherworldly backdrop all to themselves.

"It's like another planet," Jessica recalled. "As you drive east from Orange County, the landscape slowly changes, and then you get there and start wondering where you are. We visited right after Thanksgiving. Barely anybody was there. We stayed for three or four nights, walking around from scenic place to scenic place. We'd find a stack of rocks we could climb; we'd meditate, do some asana, take pictures. It was amazing. Totally free-form. I never thought a place like this existed. You don't have to be a professional climber or experienced camper. You can just wander around and do yoga on the rocks."

Although formal, structured yoga retreats typically enact a schedule of attuning your body with the rising and setting of the sun, the benefit of practicing without any barrier between you and nature is that nature itself often becomes the teacher. "When you're camping in a space with nobody else around and no lights, you naturally wake up with the sun," Jessica continued. "We practiced sun salutations with the sun actually rising. It's powerful. That fresh cold air in your lungs, on your skin. Looking at the silhouette of the Joshua trees and the mountains and the sun. You feel connected. In the morning I began to think, *I am part of this, this is part of me.* You have this sense that god is in you. You are love! This is when I realized I wanted to be a yoga teacher. All of a sudden, I got what people were talking about—why people want to get up and hike and stay connected in nature."

Whether visitors choose to engage the structure of a group retreat or wander into the expanse with nothing but a sleeping bag and a water canteen, they will be rewarded by revelations from the quiet, stark intimacy of this famous desert. "Joshua Tree is such a different place from where so many people live," Jessica said. "It's a perfect place to reset, refresh, tap back into your true nature, reflect on your goals; it's a perfect place for a self-retreat. LA is wonderful, but it also has traffic and trash. It's easy to get lost in the shuffle of day-to-day life. It's important for us spiritual beings to forge a space, one that isn't cost or time prohibitive, where you can connect with nature and reconnect with yourself, your goals, and who you are. People say you should travel to flip your perspective, and I agree with this. We can't all get a flight to Bali, but we can all get a tent."

JESSICA RIHAL is a Los Angeles–based plus-size yoga instructor (200-HR) and a strong advocate of fitness/wellness for all bodies. In addition to teaching at Everybody Los Angeles and Curvy Love Fit Hub, she co-hosts the Garden of Edyn podcast, which aims to create a conversation surrounding wellness, joyful movement, and life as plus-size WOC. She believes that all bodies can be and deserve to be celebrated through movement and enjoys doing so by teaching students how to adapt yoga to the body they're in today with no "end goal." Through yoga, Jessica has been able to reconnect with her own body and has discovered her passion for movement and exercise for the pure joy of it. As well, she is dedicated to helping others rebuild and redefine their connection to movement and exercise.

If You Go

▶ **Getting There**: The closest airports are Palm Springs (forty-five minutes away by car) or Ontario International (1.5 hours away by car), although Los Angeles (three hours away by car) has more flight options. From any airport, Joshua Tree National Park is best reached by car. Most major roads in the park are paved.

▶ **Best Time to Visit**: Joshua Tree is a national park, open year-round. Spring sees the best temperatures and famous desert blooms, nurtured by occasional showers. Summer, although peak tourist season, sees daily temperatures regularly over 100 degrees Fahrenheit; preparations for extreme heat are recommended.

▶ **Accommodations**: Many campsites in the park can be reserved at nps.gov/jotr. A list of hotels in the small town of Joshua Tree can be found with the Joshua Tree Visitors Guide at joshuatree.guide.

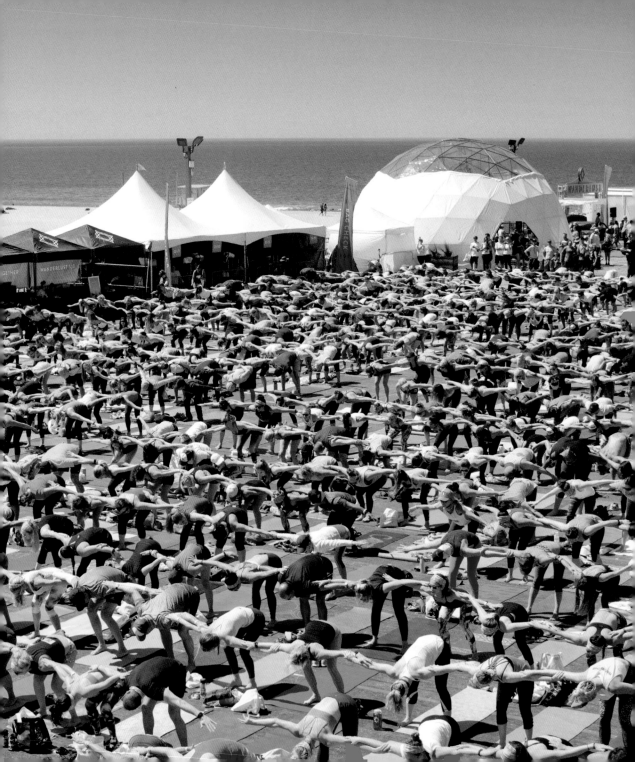

LOS ANGELES

RECOMMENDED BY **Felicia Tomasko**

"I'm a reluctant Angeleno," began Felicia Tomasko. "I love Los Angeles, but I didn't think I would love it. Originally, I moved here for a relationship, but I stayed because of the yoga. The spectrum of what you can do in LA is much bigger than anywhere else. When you apply that ethos to fitness and wellness and yoga and spirituality it goes beyond 'trends.' This is experimentation. You are setting trends. Things that spread around the world start here."

Los Angeles is the launchpad from which the rocket ship of yoga soared into the Western world. Paramahansa Yogananda, the superstar guru widely credited as the man who brought yoga from India to the West, founded the international headquarters of his Self-Realization Fellowship there in the 1920s. A noted world traveler, the kriya yoga monk referred to Los Angeles as the most spiritual city in the entire United States, dubbing it the "Benares of America." (Benares is the holiest of the seven sacred cities in India.) Perhaps it was the calm, dry air, or the magic of a city of eternal sunshine, suspended between the ocean and the mountains. At any rate, Yogananda, and numerous gurus of various lineages who followed thereafter, cemented the town's reputation as the prime headquarters for the processing and circulation of yogic teachings in the West. "It's been over a hundred years; so many great teachers have converged in LA," Felicia added. "It really is a place for spiritual awakening and spiritual connection."

For visitors, the trouble is not in finding a studio, but rather narrowing down your list of potentials. "This is the city that eats, breathes, and sleeps yoga," Felicia added. "Even if you don't intend on going to a yoga class, you might bump into one." The city that is perpetually 72 degrees Fahrenheit and sunny offers, above all, a unique ability to practice yoga outside virtually year-round. "There's a sense of really integrating yoga with the

OPPOSITE:
LA is considered
the birthplace of
yoga in America,
and yogis
regularly take
over the famous
Santa Monica
Pier during
festivals.

natural world," Felicia said. "LA is often seen as a sprawling city of cars, but there's a tight relationship with the great outdoors here, so there are plenty of places to practice outside. The Santa Monica Pier, for example—one of the top-five most Instagrammable spots to do yoga in the world—has a free yoga series. You can even go out and *do* yoga on a paddleboard any time of the year. Just a short walk down from the pier, Venice Beach, with its rollerbladers and hippie vibes, hosts countless yoga classes on the warm sand and along the bike path. Inland from the Pacific, Runyon Canyon, Los Angeles' 160-acre outdoor park, welcomes downward dogs amid sagebrush and birds'-eye views of the vast cityscape below. "Even downtown, you can go to Skyspace and do yoga at the top of a skyscraper, as if you're in the sky," Felicia continued.

"One of the most amazing moments for me was on the Santa Monica Pier, where you're literally practicing over the Pacific Ocean. An entire school of dolphins came by while we were doing an asana. Another time, there was a series of migrating whales that came into viewing distance of the pier. Everyone just stopped. It was mid–yoga practice. LA isn't normally a whale-watching place, so to be able to see that in the midst of a city was such a reminder that we are always part of the natural world, and we practice in community with it."

Aside from an embarrassment of riches in free outdoor yoga venues, visitors can enjoy all manner of creative and experimental yoga practices indoors. Nude yoga, Christian yoga, brew yoga, yoga raves, and even black metal yoga are all on the menu for you to sample. "Museums have yoga. The Getty has yoga. There's even a cat café that socializes rescue pets, and people can do yoga with the cats, helping them get used to having humans around," Felicia recalled. "UCLA has free meditation sessions, recorded live at the Hammer Museum on campus. It's on Thursdays. And that's free too. You can just show up."

After trying every yoga variation known to man, visitors can enjoy a wealth of yoga history sites across the area. In the Pacific Palisades, an affluent enclave of marble stairs and serpentine roads that are surrounded by high grassy cliffs overlooking the sparkling Pacific, Paramahansa Yogananda's Self-Realization Fellowship Headquarters welcomes all visitors to the jewel green lake shrine dedicated to the guru himself. "It's one of my favorite places to go and to take people from out of town," Felicia enthused. "It's an odd mashup of things: It has a windmill from Holland, some of Mahatma Gandhi's ashes, a pair of swans. It has a very oasis type of feel. You don't necessarily go there for an asana practice, but you can meditate and just be present. And it's completely free. You see lots of couples wandering around on first dates; it's a well-known cheap date spot.

"Sometimes people call LA superficial. But it's also a place of exploration and depth—you can do just about anything and be anyone and be accepted. LA is a home for people to express their creativity, and the creativity and ethos of the city spreads everywhere, especially into the yoga scene. You see it everywhere—on outdoor patios, at museums, on the beach. People practice yoga with their kids and their families. Some people come with their dogs. These are the images that stick out to me when I think about Los Angeles. People of all different backgrounds and walks of life are out, practicing yoga, together. Everywhere."

FELICIA TOMASKO is an E-RYT-500, C-IAYT, YACEP, and CAP certified yoga instructor, with an active private practice in both yoga and Ayurveda. In addition to being a registered nurse, she is the former president of the California Association of Ayurvedic Medicine and served for nine years on the board of directors of the National Ayurvedic Medical Association and the Academic Collaboration for Integrative Health. Felicia is an active member of the yoga therapy community and teaches on the faculty of the Yoga Studies Extension Program and the Yoga Therapy RX Program at Loyola Marymount University. A trained Ayurvedic chef, she is a former faculty member at the Natural Epicurean, specializing in food as medicine and Ayurvedic theory. In 2002, Felicia was part of the team that founded *LA YOGA Magazine*, where she is the current editor-in-chief, and she is the editorial director at Bliss Network.

If You Go

▶ **Getting There**: Los Angeles International is a major hub for many airlines. Public transportation in the city is not known for its efficiency, however. It's best to rent a car or take a taxi from the airport into the city.

▶ **Best Time to Visit**: The city of perpetual sunny skies doesn't really have a bad season, although summer temperatures often climb over 90 degrees Fahrenheit. Spring sees lovely blooms and occasional showers.

▶ **Accommodations**: In such a massive city, there's an accommodation for every budget and lifestyle. The Los Angeles Tourism & Convention Board lists several at discover losangeles.com.

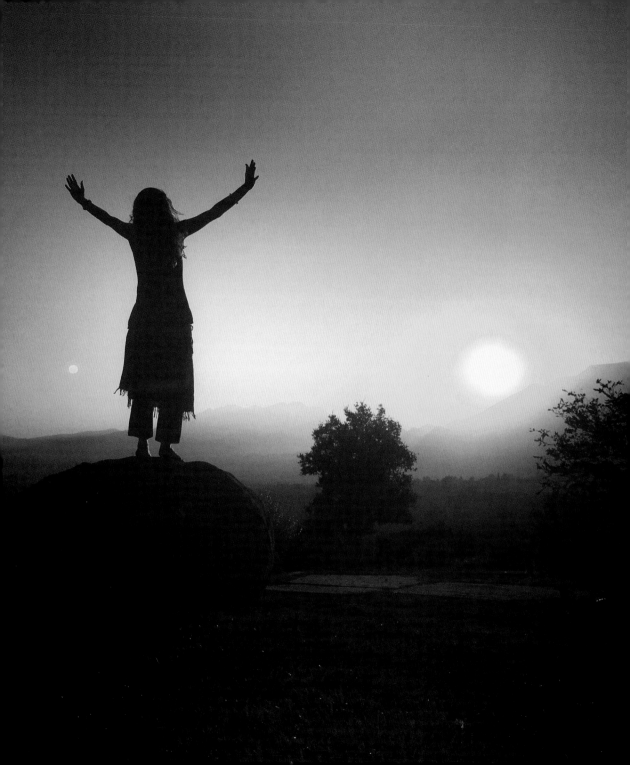

OJAI

RECOMMENDED BY **Serge Bandura**

From any angle, Ojai has a well-earned reputation as a refuge. Located in a green valley under the ruddy, striped bluffs of Southern California's Topa Topa Mountains (many of which are considered power spots for the Chumash), you would have trouble finding Ojai unless someone told you about it. However, the picturesque adobe arches, open café patios, lush native flowers spilling out of every park, and proud history have prevented Ojai from staying anyone's secret.

"It's a place of great natural beauty, great creativity, and spiritualism," began Serge Bandura. "The first time I came to Ojai, I was visiting an Indian teacher of mine, Uma Inder, who herself had traveled from abroad in order to teach there. I then completed several advanced yoga trainings with other local teachers in town and eventually went on to begin teaching and producing my own music events."

Ojai has long cultivated itself as a place where local art, peaceful counterculture, and spiritual retreats can flourish. The twentieth-century philosopher and spiritual leader Jiddu Krishnamurti has probably had the most impact on the city, settling in the valley in 1928 and operating what some skeptics described as a cult. A school in his honor still runs today, educating children on principles of environmentalism, tolerance, and the importance of a global outlook. The hills around Ojai may be covered in the remnants of other communes past, but this may largely go unnoticed by weekend vacationers. The downtown is ready to greet visitors with luxurious spas, yoga shalas, and vegetarian eateries. Even the street corners seem to be crafted with intention (it is a city of artists, after all).

Despite its notoriety as a tourist town, visitors who stay past the weekend will quickly see past the boutique shops and experience Ojai's most quintessential characteristic: its ironclad sense of community.

OPPOSITE:
A joyful yogi
pauses and
honors the sun
as night takes
hold in Ojai.

"I had two friends in the local Ojai community who kept asking me to open a studio here," continued Serge. "It had never been my intention, and at first I thought, *No, it's not needed*, but they just kept nudging me. There were other studios in Ojai already; I wasn't sure I needed to start another. Then, one day, I was taking a walk down the main drag and bumped into CJ, who operated an auto garage downtown for thirty years. I asked him offhand if it was for rent, and he immediately said, 'Yes, it is.' I came and sat with him, and we talked. It had actually been on the market for a year and a half. He'd been getting the runaround from several people. So I saw this as a way I could create a community space with and for my friends, and also help this special man who had been in Ojai for sixty years move into his next phase of life. Yoga is about cultivating union in ourselves and in our communities. It felt synchronistic, an alignment of so many different things."

Ojai's spirituality is frequently connected with its landscape, from Jiddu Krishnamurti seeing an angelic presence over the Topa Topas to the ley lines that are reputed to run through the valley. A natural phenomenon that enchants residents and tourists alike is the "Pink Moment," the light of sunset that causes the six-thousand-foot bluffs surrounding the valley to flash a divine pink. "I had a moment at Meditation Mount years ago," reflected Serge. "There was a large group of people gathered in the gardens to watch the sunset, and everyone fell completely silent. It was like this unspoken agreement that it was a moment of sanctuary. And I thought, *What is so meaningful about this experience that everyone is feeling, what is making this moment happen?* Immediately I realized 'light and space,' and it struck me as a concept: When those two things come together, something happens in the human soul. That's why our studio is made of glass, to make way for tremendous amounts of light to pour in from the mountains. When we have this experience on an external level, it does something to us; we begin to feel it internally; we transfer that feeling of light and space into ourselves. And that's one thing that's always been so powerful about Ojai, the ability to retreat into the mountains and commune with that light and space."

In 2017, the Thomas Fire brought Ojai to its knees, turning the guardian mountains into walls of fire, completely encircling the town. Many lost their homes, and citizens fled as refugees. Ojai suffered a tremendous loss. And yet, its spirit survived and strengthened, and today it's bursting with as much life as ever.

"Ojai is a gem," concluded Serge. "As it expands and grows, I'd like to give a reminder to anyone who is visiting there to honor the Chumash peoples who walked there for thousands and thousands of years before us and to respect the locals who have been struggling to maintain their way of life as the town grows. We're here to honor all those who paved the way for the community we continue to build in this beautiful valley we call home."

SERGE BANDURA entered residential training in a tantric yoga school as a homeless nineteen-year-old, completing a thousand-hour yoga teacher training program in traditional lineage-based hatha yoga. He continued his studies in kundalini yoga, Taoist yoga, Tibetan yoga, and Sufism with a number of sages in the United States and eventually on the Indian subcontinent. He went on to complete more than twenty retreats with Pema Khandro Rinpoche, wisdom holder and lama in the Nyingma school of Tibetan Buddhism. He further took refuge and continues to honor/attend teachings with Lama Acharya Dawa Chhodak Rinpoche, and spent years studying and practicing traditional kundalini tantra intensively with Umaa (Uma Inder). He holds a BA in religious studies with an emphasis on South Asian traditions, a certificate in yoga philosophy, a diploma in the study of yoga and Ayurveda, and an E-RYT 500 designation from the Yoga Alliance. Serge refined his studies in Sanskrit mantra with Vedic priest and pujari Shri Shivakumar and study of sacred texts with Srivatsa Ramaswami. He also feels blessed to call Saul David Raye one of his most important teachers. Today, he is the owner of Light and Space yoga studio in Ojai and produces music under the moniker Earthtones.

If You Go

▶ **Getting There**: Most people fly into Los Angeles International Airport, a major hub served by hundreds of carriers, and then rent a car for the two-hour drive into the mountains. A shuttle can also be chartered from the airport with advance notice.
▶ **Best Time to Visit**: Ojai has wonderful spring blooms and hot summers. It is sunny year-round.
▶ **Accommodations**: Ojai has upscale resorts and boutique hotels, explorable at ojai visitors.com.

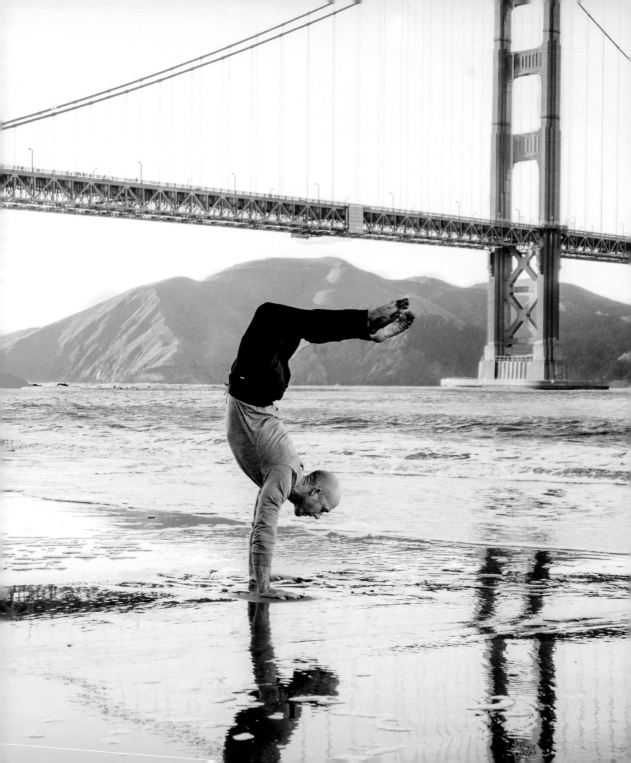

SAN FRANCISCO

RECOMMENDED BY **Zoey Gold**

"If San Francisco was a person, that person would do yoga," began Zoey Gold.

Although Los Angeles holds the honor of being ground zero for yoga in the West, in no other place did the message have such resonance as in San Francisco. The foggy city began its favorite hobby in the mid-1950s, with the first yoga studio opening by Walt and Magana Baptiste. It was inspired by Vivekananda, the swami who first spoke to Americans about yoga at the World Parliament of Religions in Chicago in 1893, and Paramahansa Yogananda, the guru who established the West's first physical yoga center in Los Angeles in 1920. Through the 1950s, '60s, and '70s, San Francisco was the epicenter of the global hippie movement, whose bohemian messages of peace, freedom, and love were directly influenced by the famous yogis and guru disciples who visited the city. In 1975, San Francisco saw the founding of America's first yoga organization, the California Yoga Teachers Association, which published the first edition of *Yoga Journal*, the West's first yoga magazine. In 2014, San Francisco's Asian Art Museum debuted "Yoga: The Art of Transformation," the world's first comprehensive art exhibit on yoga's history. Put simply, this city likes its flow.

From posh Nob Hill to the quirky Mission to techie SoMa, nearly every San Franciscan you bump into has taken at least a handful of classes and will probably be ready to tell you all about their favorite studios. The defining feature of San Francisco's yoga scene is its lack of ego. "What makes San Francisco so special is this community," Zoey continued. "You don't get this in any other city. I see familiar faces in almost every class I go to, regardless of the studio. There are people I've seen in class twelve times, or showered next to eleven times, and then one of you says hi and you're getting a drink. It's fun. There isn't that 'holier than thou' hierarchy; everyone has their unique personal goals, but the

OPPOSITE:
In the city that eats, sleeps, and breathes yoga, San Franciscans practice both indoors and out.

DESTINATION 15

community feels even. I used to work for CorePower as a cleaner, and the teachers never looked down on me. It's extremely safe to experiment and be yourself here. Not necessarily in a way that other places aren't, but it stands out to me as the defining feature. This is the first place where I've ever worked out in a sports bra. Whereas in Minnesota, where I'm from, people would be staring at me."

From gold chasers to tie-dyed war protestors to start-up dreamers, San Fransisco is known for its pioneer spirit. Blending that spirit with yoga results in a city full of far more than just the traditional shala offering. "There is so much variety," reflected Zoey. "It's hard to even know where to start. The other day I walked into a studio and it was 'Lizzo versus Beyoncé day' and we were all jamming out. There's the more serious Yoga Tree, which is great for varied ages and abilities; they really help you understand what level you're at, so you don't have to guess if something is going to be too hard or too easy. Love Story Yoga in the Mission is also wonderful. It's heated, with about a hundred people in each class and wood floors that creak. You have to commit to two hours of class, but, if you allow yourself the space, you feel refreshed in a way you've never felt before. Then, of course, there's CorePower, which is my home base. It's more workout oriented, but they offer things like glow-in-the-dark yoga, where everyone wears necklaces and they turn black lights on. They did this for Halloween and played 'The Monster Mash' and 'Thriller.' The lines for these classes are out the door."

Beyond the studio, San Franciscans take advantage of their temperate climate by laying out their mats in the outdoors. Every year on June 21, to celebrate the International Day of Yoga, large crowds move through postures together at San Francisco's Marina Green. Sunset yoga at Baker Beach, the birthplace of Burning Man, is a regular weeknight affair, occasionally featuring silent disco headphones. OutdoorYoga SF offers "Soulflow," where a mass of yogis gather under blue and purple stage lights in the Palace of Fine Arts for a collective flow. You can even downward dog under the cool stone arches inside Grace Cathedral, the seat of the Episcopal Diocese of California.

Walking through the skyscrapers and wind-tunneled corridors of the downtown Financial District, visitors might be surprised to find the streets lined with as many yoga studios as banks and tech employees dashing about with rolled mats slung over one shoulder, heading in for a quick class on lunch break. "The bottom line is that it's not intimidating," concluded Zoey. "I know there exists this idea that San Francisco is superficial, but the community is real and so are the people. It's so safe, and so strong. When I ask friends to come with me to a class, they might say, 'Oh, I'm not good at yoga, I can't do that,' and I always say, 'I wish I could show you how little that matters.' I feel that way at all of these studios. There's never a time when I think that I don't belong or that the flow is too hard. I failed my first teacher training twice before I passed, but everyone at the studio was encouraging and didn't let me get down on myself. There is a big acknowledgment here that everyone is just human. That's the real culture."

ZOEY GOLD lives and works in San Francisco as a sculpt yoga teacher at CorePower SF and manager at a start-up. She is a transplant from the Midwest and was a student of CorePower Yoga for twelve years before gaining her teacher certification in San Francisco in 2019. Previously, she was a student wellness advocate at Carleton College and an education and outreach manager at Planned Parenthood. Her passion for public health and individual wellness has inspired her to travel across the world to practice and learn from different cultures and experts.

If You Go

▶ **Getting There**: San Francisco is served by most major carriers. From the airport, the light rail system BART will take you into the heart of the city.

▶ **Best Time to Visit**: May through August, the typical tourist season, tends to be cool and pleasant, but the Bay Area experiences a strong second summer, with temperatures often going up in September and October.

▶ **Accommodations**: Options range from the emblematic Fairmont Nob Hill (415-772-5000; fairmont.com) to the quirky, budget-friendly Adelaide hostel in Union Square (415-359-1915; adelaidehostel.com). A fuller list of hotels can be found with the San Francisco Travel Association at sftravel.com.

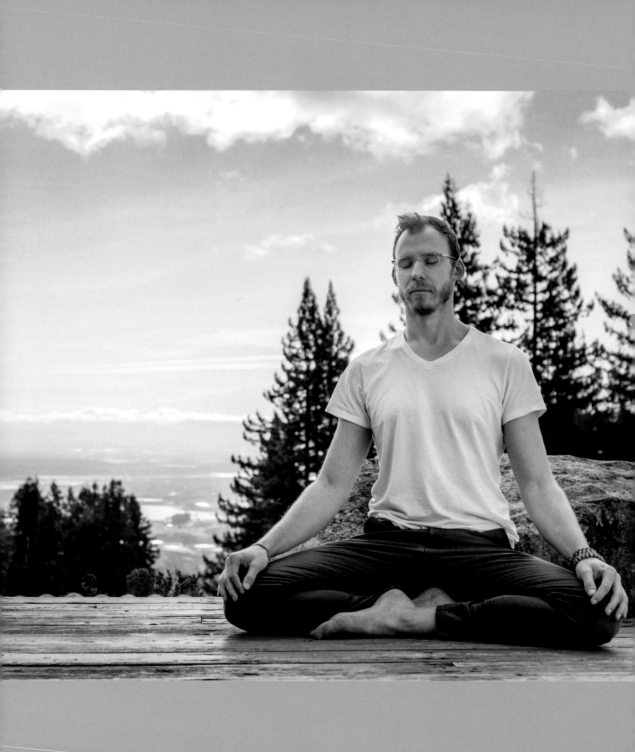

WATSONVILLE

RECOMMENDED BY **Broderick Rodell**

Broderick Rodell began practicing yoga seriously in 2009. It was a trip to Mount Madonna that truly cemented his calling.

"I'm an intense person, so when I decided to focus on yoga, I explored all of the available possibilities," he shared. "In 2009, I was at an event center in New York helping facilitate their summer retreats. I met a woman there who recommended Mount Madonna Center. I think she saw my passion, that I wanted to pursue this 100 percent. She added that I looked a bit like the guru there, as I had dreadlocks and a beard. 'I think it will resonate with you, the holistic nature of the place.'

"When I reached Mount Madonna the following year, I got into a much more detailed study of yoga. They offer a classical perspective with a focus on the eight limbs. But the teaching is not full-on traditional or dogmatic. Though an Indian guru—Baba Hari Dass—started the place, it has an American flavor. Initially, I went for a three-month starter program. I went back later and stayed for a year, continuing my study."

Mount Madonna Center is nestled in the southern end of the Santa Cruz Mountains above the small city of Watsonville, one of California's most productive agricultural areas. (The region is one of America's top strawberry producers.) The serene mountains here are a far cry from the frenzied pace of Silicon Valley, just an hour to the north. Here the tempo more closely mirrors the gradual progress of the banana slug (one of the region's denizens, and the mascot of nearby University of California, Santa Cruz) and the inexorable upward yearning of the old-growth redwoods. Black-tailed deer, black bears, bobcats, and cougars also make these mountains home. "The property at Mount Madonna is really quite lovely," Broderick continued. "They have over three hundred acres, and you're up high enough that you have a view over Watsonville and to the east over the San

OPPOSITE:
Mount Madonna
offers an island
of serenity near
the hubbub of
Silicon Valley.

16

DESTINATION

Francisco Bay. There are some beautiful stands of redwoods. The hiking opportunities available at Mount Madonna add to the overall experience."

Though he left this life in 2018, Baba Hari Dass—known affectionately as Babaji by the many who knew and practiced with him—is very much alive at Mount Madonna. Born near Almora, India, in 1923, he left his family at just eight years old to begin his yogic studies. When he turned twenty-nine, Babaji took an initial twelve-year vow of silence. However, this seemed to bring him such great peace and inner silence that, once twelve years had passed, he remained silent another fifty-four years until his death. After completing the traditional vows of a *Vairagi Vaishnav*—a level of achievement in Vaishnavism—Babaji had the classical grounding to teach Yoga Sutras of Patanjali, Bhagavad Gita, and Samkhya Karika as well as the philosophy and practices of ashtanga yoga, karma yoga, bhakti yoga, jnana yoga, and tantra yoga. He first came to America in 1971, and in 1978 he inspired the founding of Mount Madonna; his teachings also inspired centers in Vancouver Island, Toronto, and Los Angeles. His mantra for living a good life was "Work honestly, meditate every day, meet people without fear, and play."

"By the time I first started visiting Mount Madonna, Babaji wasn't living there, but he'd be present two days a week," Broderick recalled. "I'm a little leery of the idea of a guru and a little introverted, so I was a bit hesitant to interact. But I didn't get a weird 'serve me' sort of vibe at all. I came away thinking that he was a sweet, kind, and generous man. His self-discipline was inspiring."

There are many ways a guest can experience the centering spirit of Mount Madonna. Retreats (ranging from weekends to several weeks or more) are held throughout the year by visiting yogis. Alternately, one can book a personal retreat and participate in yoga practice, spiritual and personal development programs, and a variety of other classes and workshops. A number of lodging options are available, including rooms in the hotel-style structures with either private or shared bathrooms; rustic cabins (with separate bathing facilities); and campsites (bring your own tent or use one of Mount Madonna's). Day passes are also offered should you only have limited time for replenishment. Nurturing vegetarian meals are served for all guests and vegan options are available. Those on a personal retreat are welcome to participate in morning yoga classes, which blend pranayama, dhyana, and asana practices. Guests may also attend any classes based on the study of classical Indian texts, like the Bhagavad Gita. Discussions are based on Babaji's commentary from decades of study and are designed to make the Indian scriptures more accessible to Westerners. Many guests will also visit the Hanumān Temple to participate in the *Ārati* devotional service, which is performed at sunrise and sunset each day.

Whatever activities you participate in, Mount Madonna's core practice of karma yoga, which Babaji defined as "union with God through service," is ever-present. A community of roughly eighty people reside at the center, working on a variety of projects. Guests are welcome to join in.

Broderick Rodell has conducted scores of retreats since studying at Mount Madonna in 2010. In 2019, he was able to return to lead his own retreat there, a bit of karma in action.

BRODERICK RODELL received his teacher training under the guidance of master Yogi Baba Hari Dass, who founded the Mount Madonna Center in the Santa Cruz Mountains of Watsonville, CA. His vision is to create educational systems and curricula that support the individual evolution toward a more whole, loving self. Broderick's approach emphasizes an integration of the whole person, incorporating tools that support the development of mind, body, and soul. In his yoga classes, workshops, trainings, and retreats, he incorporates knowledge gathered from the Western sciences of psychology, physiology, and anatomy to complement the rich yogic science from India. Broderick also holds a PhD in chemical engineering from the Georgia Institute of Technology and a doctor of naturopathic medicine (ND) degree from Bastyr University. Based in the San Francisco Bay Area, he leads classes there and retreats at Mount Madonna Center and beyond. Learn more about his practice at yogawithbroderick.com.

If You Go

▶ **Getting There**: Most visitors fly to San Jose International Airport, which is served by many carriers. Mount Madonna Center is in Watsonville, roughly fifty miles south of the airport.

▶ **Best Time to Visit**: Mount Madonna welcomes visitors throughout the year. Watsonville has a mild Mediterranean climate, though winters see more rain than the rest of the year.

▶ **Accommodations**: Mount Madonna (408-847-0406; mountmadonna.org) offers a number of different lodging options, as well as day passes.

16

DESTINATION

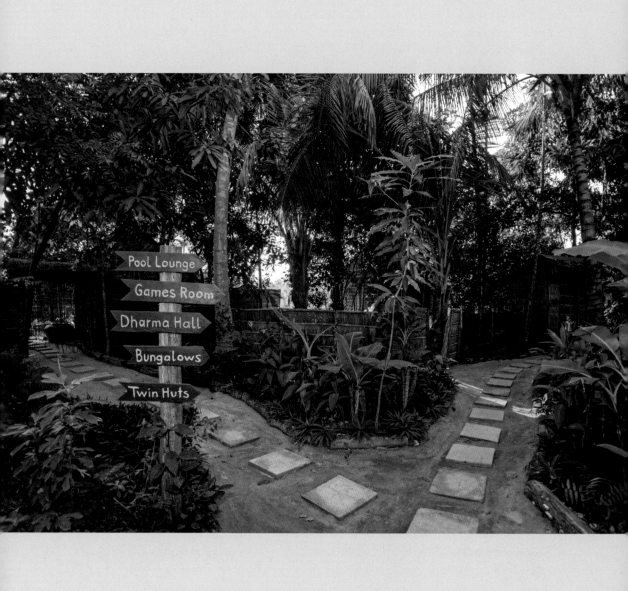

SIEM REAP

RECOMMENDED BY **Joel Altman**

Puravi Joshi, the famous London banker turned yoga teacher, calls Cambodia one of the most peaceful, safe places to practice yoga. While perhaps most famous for its ancient Hindu temples, especially Angkor Wat, this South Asian country offers a rich tapestry of ancient Buddhist and Hindu philosophy, modern monks, notoriously friendly citizens, and spiritual vacationers. With an emphasis on cultivating the inner mind, yogis looking for an intensive practice can immerse themselves at the Hariharalaya Yoga & Meditation Retreat Center in Siem Reap. "The name is from the ancient capital of the Khmer Empire, which is where we're located," began Joel Altman. "Now it's a traditional Cambodian farming village. With its thatched huts and temples set in the jungle, it's almost like a camp. Simplicity is important to us. I think of it like an adult playground, where people are encouraged to be playful and creative."

Yoga in Cambodia is hardly new. Many scholars claim the country was practicing and embracing yogic philosophy even before the Hindu Khmer Empire, which ran from roughly 800 CE to the mid-fifteenth century. This rich history is no doubt why nearly every yogi who visits the country comes back extolling its virtues. "I embarked on the spiritual path twenty-one years ago," reflected Joel. "I was living in ashrams in Canada and Brazil, then India. I never had any intention to start a center. Then I got sick and robbed in Thailand, and a friend said, 'Come see me in Cambodia.' I did a personal meditation retreat with some elder Buddhist monks here, and I came out of it with a vision for a grassroots community learning center to help people get back in touch with the creative flow of life. And here we are ten years later."

Set among two acres of lush jungle in the shade of the temples of Angkor, Hariharalaya is a picture-perfect slice of Cambodian beauty. "Every direction you look is filled with

OPPOSITE:
The greenery
of Cambodia
abounds at
every turn.

plants," Joel continued. "We have more than twenty varieties of fruiting trees—mango, jackfruit, coconut, custard apple, banana—and thirty hammocks strung throughout the property where you can go rest and sway with the trees."

Many yogis who travel the world to deepen their expertise may expect to pay a pretty penny for the opportunity. However, Hariharalaya flips this expectation on its head. "We do student training programs, as opposed to a teacher training program," said Joel with a laugh. "Our goal is to help you learn to be a student of life, a student of yourself. The main focus is not what happens on the mat, but how we live our life moment to moment. It's not about getting into that complicated pose but getting into that center." Many visitors may do double takes at the price tag, which is half to one quarter of a standard English-language South Asian yoga retreat. "It's really important for us to keep it authentic and affordable," Joel added. "The yoga world needs affordable, high-quality spaces like this."

Attendees sign up for a full six days, and surrender all phones and tablets at the front desk for a full digital detox. "The program is set up for a group of twenty-six people," Joel explained. "We want to keep it intimate. A lot of teaching actually happens between classes. Your teachers share all the spaces with you. Meals, walks, games—we're always accessible and able to connect with people. Everybody is family by the first or second day."

During the six-day program, mornings begin at six A.M. with the ringing of a gong. Attendees gather for a practice that focuses on postures, breathing, meditation, and, occasionally, chanting. Breakfast follows in silence. "We believe a lot in silence here," Joel said. "In the evening, between 10:30 P.M. and waking up, we have general silence. The fourth day is a full day of silence. We have a spa and lots of massage and Ayurvedic treatments, but this is a place to be challenged, rather than pampered, to really go deep."

Going deep does not mean going dull, however. With respect to the inner journey, Hariharalaya displays much of the playfulness that Cambodian culture is known for. "We do a lot of laughter yoga, which is so wonderful: to see people awakening the inner child and smiling for no reason. It's pure, pure joy," Joel enthused. "Or you catch people jumping on the trampoline, giving that pure laughter from the heart. The jungle juice bar in the center of the place is my favorite; all of our juice is fresh from the trees around us. One night we have a local Khmer wedding band come, and the kids from the village teach us to dance. On the last day, we invite monks from the local village to perform a traditional water blessing."

When the program is done, visitors are encouraged to wander out into the remains of the ancient capital and take in the area's incredible treasures. Nearby Bakong Temple, a predecessor to Angkor Wat, is an architectural wonder, the first temple mountain of sandstone constructed by the Khmer Empire. "The proportions are unbelievable," reflected Joel. "It's a huge temple, surrounded by a massive moat. It's like the pyramids of Giza.

"Cambodia is a great place to go deep with yourself. Almost everyone who comes to Hariharalaya is new to yoga. It's a place where people feel they can connect and open themselves in ways they haven't for many years. Cambodia is full of natural joy and pure hearts; it's such an inspiring place for this."

JOEL ALTMAN is a mystic, polyglot, yogi, vegan chef, poet, classical musician, jeweler, and lover of life. Joel was first initiated in a traditional kriya yoga path in 2000. He met his gurus Sri Karunamayi, Sri Shivabalayogi, and Sri Amritanandamayi Ma around 2005, and spent years studying integral yoga and absorbing the wisdom of Being from the presence of many great saints, sages, and enlightened masters. Before arriving in Cambodia, Joel studied at ashrams in India, Brazil, Quebec, and the United States. Since 2010 he has dedicated his time and energy to maintaining the Hariharalaya Center in Siem Reap as an authentic space to explore and experience this great joy and freedom of awakening through integral yoga, conscious living, community, and creativity. His book of dharma talks, *The Foundations of Stillness*, was published in 2013.

If You Go

▶ **Getting There**: Fly into Siem Reap, which connects through most major cities throughout Asia and is served by Lanmei Airlines (+855 93822999; lanmeiairlines.com) and Sky Angkor Airlines (+855 23217130; skyangkorair.com). From there, grab a taxi or a tuktuk for the hour drive to Hariharalaya.
▶ **Best Time to Visit**: December through January is the sunny and dry season for Cambodia. April and May are the hottest and most humid months, and from June through November you can expect drenching monsoon rains (but fewer crowds).
▶ **Accommodations**: Hariharalaya is bookable at.hariharalaya.com.

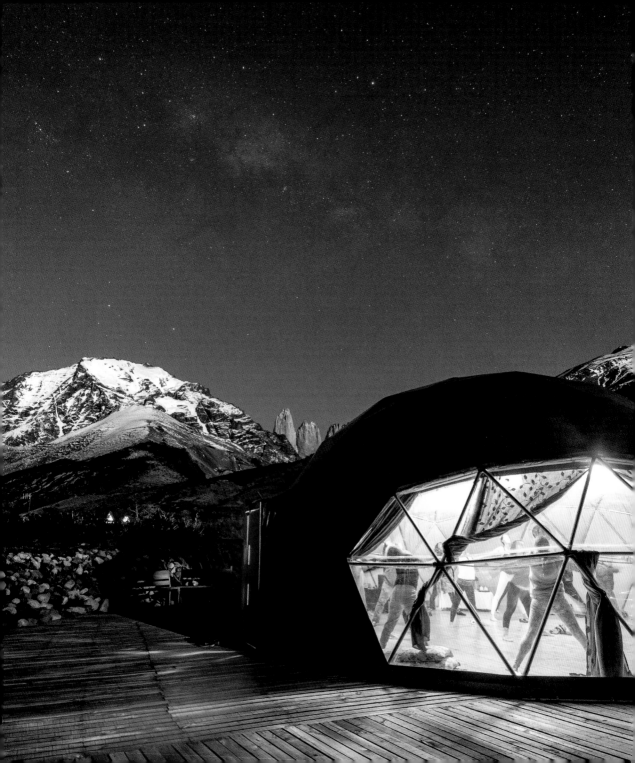

TORRES DEL PAINE NATIONAL PARK

RECOMMENDED BY **Sandra Tedeschi**

It was a quest to explore the "power of place" that first brought Sandra Tedeschi to Patagonia. "I was living in Costa Rica at the time—2008—where I was running trips that combined adventure, travel, and yoga. Costa Rica was a popular ecotourism destination, and travelers liked the idea of including a yoga component while on vacation. It was a chance to combine a personal journey with sightseeing. The people who came on a retreat with me in Costa Rica wanted to travel to new destinations. Chile came up as another adventure and nature wonderland. I visited Patagonia and was immediately struck by this sense of strong energy; it's a destination with what I call a power of place. It unites the five elements of nature—earth, water, fire, air, and space—in a dramatic fashion. The remoteness and vastness of the landscape, its incredible beauty, affects your being. Patagonia is one of those destinations that leaves people feeling whole and in an elated state of being. Ten years later I returned to lead adventure yoga retreats hosted at EcoCamp in Torres del Paine National Park."

Patagonia is as much a state of mind as a place. Encompassing roughly four hundred thousand square miles of seemingly endless steppes, groaning glaciers, spiky pink granite peaks, and electric-blue lakes, wind-pummeled Patagonia—divided between Chile and Argentina across the bottom of South America—is still very much a frontier. Torres del Paine National Park, at the southern tip of the Andes in the region of Magallanes, combines all the natural wonders Patagonia is known for in its 935 square miles. A number of famed trekking routes wind among the park's glaciers, lakes, and mountains, including the W Trek and the Paine Circuit. But you needn't strap on a backpack to experience the park's wonders. EcoCamp Patagonia provides a one-of-a-kind venue to use as a base camp from which to explore the park via day excursions.

OPPOSITE:
At EcoCamp,
yogis can practice
in a geodesic
dome in the
shadow of the
iconic spires of
Torres del Paine.

DESTINATION **18**

EcoCamp combines a premium location—overlooking the three iconic granitic spires of Torres del Paine (South, Central, and North) just inside the borders of the park—with the novelty of geodesic domes as living structures. EcoCamp's dome design was inspired by the Kaweskars, a group of nomadic Patagonian inhabitants who built easily dismantled semicircular huts from simple materials, leaving no trace behind. EcoCamp pioneered the use of geodesic domes for travelers in 1999. Their standard domes keep the often-fierce Patagonian wind at bay and feature ceiling windows for viewing the southern stars. Like your standard-issue tent, the standard domes lack heat, but an assortment of fleece blankets should keep you cozy. (More-ornate domes that include propane heaters and a private bathroom with a composting toilet are also available.) Guests take their meals and socialize in one of the community domes, which boast woodstoves, a bar, a library, and an "asadero" platform for the preparation of Patagonian lamb barbecues for meat-eaters. Several of the park's popular trails can be joined right from EcoCamp.

The setup at EcoCamp is phenomenal," Sandra said. "There's no town; you're just in the national park. As you drive in, there are impressive vistas of the landscape—mountains, glacial lakes, and the famous Patagonian 'pampa' (vast grassy plains). You'll often see guanacos [a small member of the camel family, resembling a llama] en route; condors and puma are also present, though less frequently encountered. On a clear day, the three towers of Los Torres are in view. While you're at EcoCamp, you're completely disconnected from the outside world. When you take the internet away, people's outlook shifts. It creates a more present connection and joyful comradery among group members."

Sandra's Patagonia retreats strive to connect visitors to the larger landscape, with yoga as an enabling component. "Each day begins with a 1.5- to 2-hour yoga session around 7:30 in the dedicated yoga dome," she described. "Each class [based around vinyasa flow] is themed on one of the five elements of nature. After breakfast, you pack your lunch and depart for the day's main activity, accompanied by EcoCamp's excellent guides. One day might be a boat tour of Grey Glacier [the south end of the Southern Patagonian Ice Field], which we embark on after driving across much of the park. Another is a hike at Laguna Azul, where guides will set up a barbecue, weather permitting. A highlight for many is making the trek to the base of Los Torres. It's fourteen miles round-trip and takes nine to ten hours. Due to the physical demands of the hike, there's lots of buildup. Not everyone is up for it. When you get to the last section of the hike, you can't see the towers. As you come over this ridge, climbing over boulders to get to the last steep push, you reach the lake that rests at the base of Los Torres. Sometimes it's cloudy, but if you arrive on a sunny day when the towers are exposed, it's a magical moment. You're fully present, tapping into the power of the place. It's the sensation you strive for in yoga practice."

At the end of the day, guests gather in one of the communal domes for happy hour. "Chile is known for its pisco sours," Sandra added. "They make these and other incredible drinks using local herbs and berries; nonalcoholic drinks are available too. Dinners are served communally, and are excellent, with many fresh salads and different types of pastas. (Grilled lamb and beef is available for meat-eaters.) This being Chile, there is as much wine on the table as there is water."

SANDRA TEDESCHI's earlier work in international humanitarian aid took her to South Asia and Africa. From her experiences in often fast-paced and high-pressured work environments, she learned the great value of a regular yoga practice to maintain balance in daily living. In 2006, Sandra changed her path and founded Vajra Sol Yoga Adventures, based in Costa Rica, which leads yoga retreats around the world. She has been practicing yoga for more than twenty-five years and currently studies under the Himalayan and tantra traditions. Sandra approaches her personal practice and the philosophy of yoga as an ever-present part of each day. On the retreats she is dedicated to facilitating and co-creating a soulful getaway for those who seek to travel deeper with yoga in a lighthearted setting.

If You Go

▶ **Getting There**: Travelers can reach Torres del Paine National Park via Punta Arenas, which is served by LAN Airlines (866-435-9526; latam.com) via Santiago.
▶ **Best Time to Visit**: Torres del Paine National Park is open year-round, though the weather is best during the austral spring and summer—October through March. Visit Vajra Sol Yoga Adventures (vajrasoltravel.com) for details about Sandra's next Patagonian retreat.
▶ **Accommodations**: EcoCamp Patagonia (800-901-6987; ecocamp.travel) offers unique camp-style lodging in geodesic domes and an array of tours around the park.

18

DESTINATION

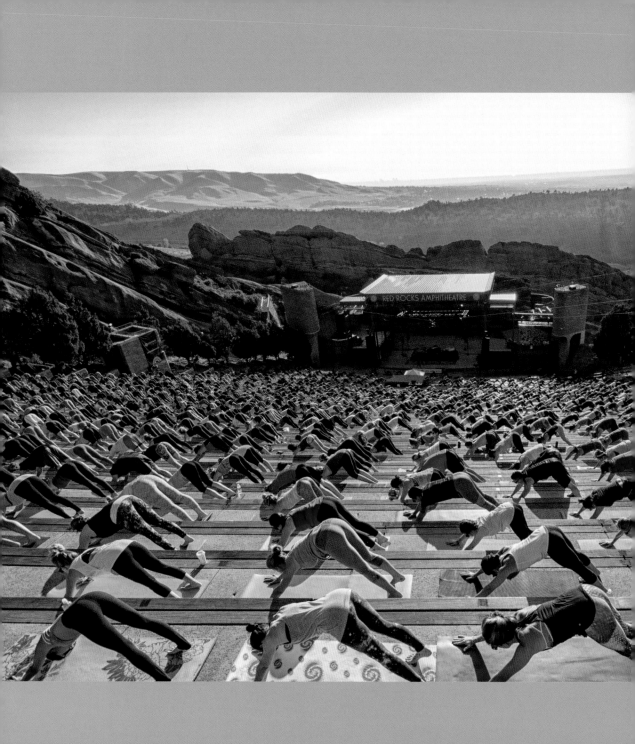

DENVER

RECOMMENDED BY **Sara Rice**

After first playing there in 1978, the Grateful Dead would go on to headline twenty shows. They've been followed by nearly every touring ensemble of note, from U2 and Dave Matthews Band to Rush and Incubus, and even John Tesh. In 2014, Sara Rice took the stage at Red Rocks, her only instruments a microphone and a yoga mat.

"Yoga on the Rocks started back in 2014," Sara began. "It's a summer activity that began with eight Saturdays over June, July, and August. They allow 2,500 people in, and the classes are generally held near sunrise, at seven A.M. You're practicing while the sun is coming up, which is pretty spectacular. And to think you're on the same stage that held acts like the Beatles and Johnny Cash is incredible! At the time I was asked to lead the class, I was teaching at the River Yoga studio and getting ready to leave for Vancouver for my work with Lululemon. Yoga on the Rocks was my last hurrah and a nice acknowledgment to my teaching and the community connections I'd built up in the area. River Yoga hosted my event." (More recently, Yoga on the Rocks offerings have expanded.)

Red Rocks rests at the transitional zone between the Great Plains and the Rockies. Anchored by two monolithic chunks of sandstone—Ship Rock to the south and Creation Rock to the north—the site sits at an elevation of 6,450 feet and has likely boasted world-class acoustics for millions of years; long before the feedback of distorted guitars rang from rock to rock, the cries of dinosaurs may have echoed here. (Each of the monoliths is believed to be more than three hundred million years old and top three hundred feet in height—taller than Niagara Falls!) Red Rocks' potential as a musical venue was first explored by an impresario named John Brisben Walker, who installed a temporary platform here in 1906 and promoted several concerts over the following years, including a performance by renowned soprano Mary Garden in 1911. A formal stage and amphitheater

OPPOSITE:
Rock and roll meets Downward Dog—that's the experience to be had at Yoga on the Rocks.

seating would be completed thirty years later, designed by Denver architect Burnham Hoyt and constructed with the help of the Civilian Conservation Corps and Works Progress Administration. Teen heartthrob Ricky Nelson is credited with playing the first "rock" show at Red Rocks in 1959. Since that time, there have been more than three thousand concerts performed here; nearly every artist will attest to the emotional, even mystical power of the place. (As of this writing, the jam band Widespread Panic has logged more shows here than anyone else, generally selling out the venue's 9,525 seats.)

What's it like to lead a yoga class at the world's most famous natural outdoor amphitheater? "For starters, there's a tunnel you pass through under the stage," Sara described. "The artists that have played at Red Rocks over the years have all signed the wall. On the stage, because of the size of the space, it's impossible to see everyone who is practicing yoga, so you have to lean in and trust the momentum of the energetic arc of the class. There's a profound spirituality just being there, a strong connection to nature. I've gone as a participant as well, and there is a wild challenge as yoga mats have to go sideways to fit on the seats. Typically, of course, you're facing the teacher—that takes some getting used to, but it's worthwhile. There's a great view of the city [which is twenty miles away], and the cool air gradually warms as the sun rises. Simply sitting at Red Rocks as the sun is rising would be a transformative experience, so doing yoga there is something profoundly spiritual."

While a session of "Yoga on the Rocks" is reason enough for many to visit Denver, the city's vibrant yoga community will keep one occupied well beyond your Saturday session. The Mile High City boasts one of America's highest concentrations of yoga studios per capita—no surprise, given that it's perennially ranked as one of the nation's healthiest cities. It wasn't always that way, though. "When I finished up as an undergrad in the late nineties, there was literally one well-known studio in Denver," Sara recalled. "We all practiced Bikram yoga; classes were busy, but you could always fit your mat in. Now, you throw a stone anywhere around Denver, and there's a yoga studio. If you were to go to a restaurant or coffee shop and ask people to hold up their hands if they do yoga, half would raise their hands. I remember seeing an ad in the early 2000s for a yogurt brand where the person holding the yogurt container was doing yoga. That's when I knew yoga had really arrived."

Denver and Boulder were home to CorePower Yoga's first studios when the company was founded in 2002, and Sara credits the brand with seeding the region with a multitude

19

DESTINATION

of strong instructors. "CorePower had three locations around Colorado when it began, and seven when I started teaching there," she recalled. "Now it has more than two hundred studios around the country. It produced so many great teachers, and many stayed in the area. Denver gives you a buffet of options, just about anything you'd want from a yoga class. If you want a hot, sweaty, nontraditional approach to yoga, one of the CorePower studios is a good bet. [There are eighteen and counting in greater Denver at this writing.] For a more traditional approach, Samadhi has several locations around the city, as one of the longest-running studios in Denver. I really love River Yoga, as they do a lot with adaptability and are very welcoming to people of all levels and abilities. Lacuna offers a different experience; they have a little juice bar and a vegan café, and offer Katonah Yoga®, which I love, as I feel like a learner again in these anatomy-focused classes."

SARA RICE rolled out a yoga mat for the first time when she was seven years old. She began teaching in 2006 at CorePower Yoga, when it had only seven locations. While her strength lies in teaching an invigorating, connected, sweaty power vinyasa flow yoga, she also holds certifications in hot yoga, restorative yoga, and sculpt yoga. She's had the opportunity to lead multiple two-hundred-hour trainings as well as focused workshops for ongoing development for teachers. When she's not leading a class at River Yoga or chasing powdery ridge lines in the Colorado Rockies with her husband, Will, and two dog pals Buzz and Brooker, Sara works at Lululemon, where she's held a variety of management positions—most recently, training and delivery manager for people and culture operations.

If You Go

▶ **Getting There**: Denver is served by most major carriers.
▶ **Best Time to Visit**: Denver attracts visitors year-round, be it for outdoor sports or the city's cultural scene. "Yoga on the Rocks" is generally held on Saturdays in June, July, and August. View the current schedule at redrocksonline.com/yoga.
▶ **Accommodations**: The Denver Convention & Visitors Bureau (800-233-6837; denver.org) lists a broad range of lodging options in the Mile High City.

19

DESTINATION

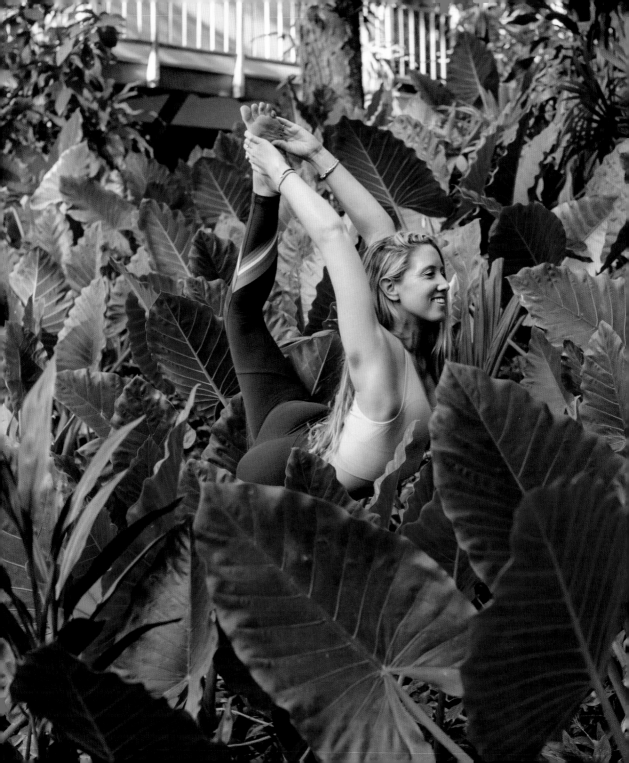

NOSARA

RECOMMENDED BY **Corey Edwards**

A pristine beach fronted by a warm and rolling Pacific. A sublime jungle setting replete with the flora and fauna that call the rainforest home. And the nexus of Costa Rica's yoga legacy, dating back almost thirty years. All of this awaits you in the village of Nosara, at Bodhi Tree.

"Nosara has a very relaxed vibe," Corey Edwards began. "It's a little beach town at the edge of the jungle that's built around yoga and surfing. Our beach is situated on the north part of the Nicoya Peninsula, and it's part of a protected refuge [the Ostional Wildlife Refuge] for nesting Olive Ridley turtles. (The turtle nesting beach, site of one of the world's largest gatherings of Olive Ridley turtles, is a bit north.) Because of the protections, no development is permitted on the beach—there are no hotels or restaurants, no people selling stuff. This keeps the area pure, raw. When people come here to do a retreat, they're not left with just a yoga hut. With the proximity of the jungle and beach, there's a life outside the yoga."

Costa Rica is much celebrated for its natural beauty, access to both the Caribbean Sea and the Pacific Ocean, and its abundance of habitat—from tropical rainforest to montane to cloud forest. It was among the first nations to recognize the possibilities of ecotourism. "Why would we cut down a tree and sell it once when we could keep it standing and sell it over and over again?" Costa Rican president Rodrigo Carazo Odio said in the early 1970s. This ethos has led to the preservation of large swaths of the country's interior (some 25 percent), and a progressive attitude toward the possibilities of ecotourism. With just .03 percent of the planet's territory, Costa Rica (the size of West Virginia) has 6 percent of the world's biodiversity. This abundance of natural wonders is certainly evident on the Nicoya Peninsula, an eighty-mile-long finger of land south of Nicaragua, in Guanacaste Province. The town of Nosara has long been on the radar of wandering surfers, offering

OPPOSITE:
In Nosara,
yogis can
practice where
the rainforest
meets the
Pacific on Costa
Rica's Nicoya
Peninsula.

consistent waves for riders of a variety of skill levels. In addition to providing healthy conditions for turtles, the peninsula seems to be amenable to human well-being: It has been designated one of the world's five "Blue Zones," regions where residents have evolved to lead healthier and longer lives.

Nosara made its way onto the destination yoga map in the early 1990s, after Don and Amba Stapleton (formerly of Kripalu Center, page 151) founded the Nosara Yoga Institute, an internationally recognized yoga teacher training center. "Years ago, my dad was traveling the world, doing yoga and surfing," Corey recalled. "He'd been impressed with Nosara, and back in 2008, he invited me to do a retreat there with him. I fell in love with the place and decided I could live there. Dad took the teacher training course and bought a house there. I was helping him out. At the time, the institute only had yoga rooms, no place for guests to stay. During trainings, students are always together; it was a hassle for people to have to leave at the end of the day. When a property became available next door, Dad bought it. Initially, we thought Don would run the operation—originally called Nosara Yoga Village—with Dad as a silent partner. But Don wanted to downsize, so he moved to the mountains. Dad made me an offer to partner with him to launch a new yoga resort. We bought out the institute property and opened Bodhi Tree Resort in 2014."

Beyond its idyllic setting, Bodhi Tree has sought to foster an environment that's welcoming to yoga neophytes and aficionados alike. "We try to place an emphasis on overall fitness, not just yoga," Corey explained. "For example, our Signature Yoga and Fitness Retreat offers pilates, weight training, and spin as well. I think this allows people who might be a little nervous to come to Costa Rica for a week of [just] yoga feel more comfortable." To that end, the resort offers a more expansive menu than some retreat centers. "We serve chicken, eggs, and fish in addition to vegan dishes," he continued. "We also try to highlight local dishes—*gallo pinto* [rice and beans, one of Costa Rica's traditional staples], fried plantains, and lots of fresh fruit. In addition to a juice bar, we have a bar that serves alcohol, should guests desire a drink. We also have local bands in on Sunday and Wednesday nights so guests can dance." Though Bodhi Tree embraces more casual yogis, yoga practice is at the resort's core. Regularly available classes include hatha, vinyasa, gentle flow, kundalini, aerial, and power yoga. The shalas look out over the jungle on to the Pacific and are open to catch the ocean breezes.

Many come to Nosara to mix yoga with a bit of surfing. "Lots of surfers incorporate yoga into their routines," Corey ventured. "There's the spiritual aspect, and the core and

DESTINATION 20

fitness component. Even if you're sitting on a board in the lineup at sunset, it's a form of meditation. You're in a magical place, with the whole horizon open to you. Even if you're too tired to surf, you can paddle out, hang on your board, and get some saltwater therapy. We get some big swells at times, though the waves are generally of a comfortable size. [Playa Marbella is more suited for experienced riders.] We operate a full surf school with lessons offered every day."

Visitors less inclined to surf can still explore the local waters. "Kayaking and standup paddleboarding are both options," Corey added. "Paddling in the mangroves, you'll see many birds and some of the other fauna Costa Rica is known for. There are several animal sanctuaries nearby, and tours can be arranged. Even walking down to the beach, you're likely to come upon armadillos, boa constrictors, and monkeys." (Three species of monkeys—white-throated capuchin, howler, and spider—are found on the peninsula.)

If you prefer to take in the surf from dry land, sunset yoga sessions on the beach are always available.

CORY EDWARDS is the manager of Bodhi Tree Resort. After spending twelve years traveling the world doing yoga and surfing with his father, Gary, he fell in love with Costa Rica, the only place he could see himself settling down. He is now in charge of all programming at Bodhi Tree and the resort's future.

If You Go

▶ **Getting There**: Liberia is the nearest international airport to Nosara and is served by several carriers, including Alaska Airlines (800-252-7522; alaskaair.com) and JetBlue (800-538-2583; jetblue.com). From here, Nosara is a roughly two-hour drive. It's about five hours' drive from San Jose, Costa Rica's largest city.

▶ **Best Time to Visit**: Bodhi Tree offers yoga classes and retreats throughout the year, though the best surf—and the driest time of the year—is from mid-December through April.

▶ **Accommodations**: Several resorts host yoga retreats in the Nosara area, including Bodhi Tree Yoga Resort (855-263-8733; bodhitreeyogaresort.com).

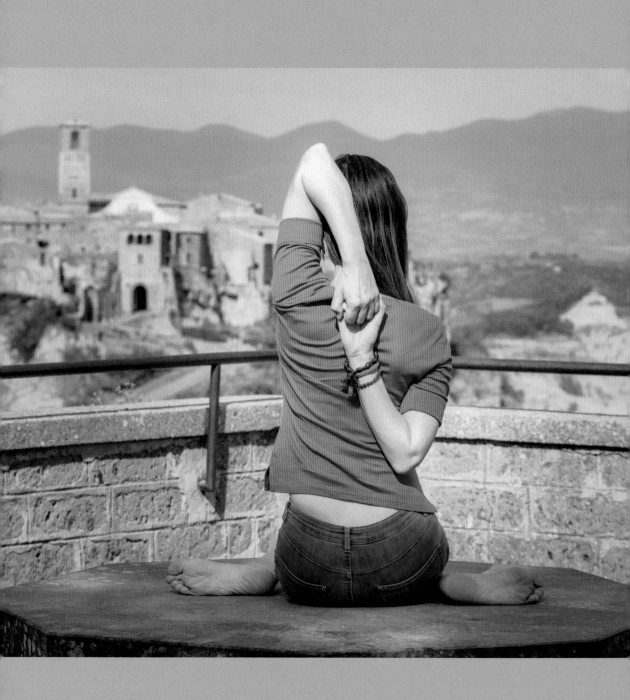

MALTA

RECOMMENDED BY **Jennifer Cortis**

"The first group doing yoga and meditation on Malta was Ananda Marga," began Jennifer Cortis, "which translates to 'path of bliss.' It's a spiritual organization, concerned with self-development. But the ashram here wasn't exactly famous. People were saying it was another religion, like a cult. Malta is a Catholic island, so there was a lot of fear at first. People had been used to going to a certain kind of church; they were used to religion, but they weren't into spirituality. That is not at all the case today, though."

The archipelago nation of Malta, just a skip down the Mediterranean from Sicily, has been inhabited since 5900 BCE. Suspended between North Africa and Europe, it has seen its fair share of cultural changes, with a history of rule by the Phoenicians, Romans, Greeks, Arabs, Normans, Aragonese, French, Spanish, and even a 150-year stint as a British colony before independence in the mid-twentieth century. There are few places in Europe with richer history, and even the landscape has a bit of an antique tinge to it, with medieval, baroque, and neoclassical architectural forms abounding in shades of ochre and ecru. Today, over 20 percent of Malta's population is foreign-born, with a particularly large representation of Brits enjoying Malta's 275 days of annual sunshine, and the kind of sea water that looks like it was imported from South Asia.

"Dada Nitya Sundaranana was my first teacher at Ananda Marga," continued Jennifer. "I went to his place for a class every weekday. It impacted my life in a very big way. No one ever told me what to do; it was all positive. I could see myself changing, organically, in a very good way, without any pressure from anyone. I was becoming happier, more balanced. I wasn't afraid to say no anymore when something bothered me. I felt I was returning to myself.

"Ananda Marga is still here, but Dada eventually left and some people asked me to teach. I kept saying no, but eventually, a year later, I felt the inspiration. I opened Lotus

OPPOSITE:
Malta's historic
landscapes and
ample ocean
bluffs offer
yogis unique
pathways
to practice
along the
Mediterranean.

DESTINATION 21

101

Room, the first actual yoga studio in Malta. We practice yoga, meditation, mantra, kirtan, sound healing, yoga trance dance, movement meditation, and we do Ayurvedic workshops. We go in depth into every subject, every chapter of yoga. I literally started with one student, and I now teach six classes per week. And it's not just us! Malta is loaded with yoga. You can find every style: ashtanga, Bikram, power yoga, vinyasa flow, yin, every class is here. We even teach the kids."

Malta may not be the only cluster of islands in the Mediterranean to attract yogis (Greece and the Amalfi Coast have gained notoriety over the past few decades), but it may be the perfect place to sample yoga in the central Mediterranean without excessive tourist crowds. Visitors can sample beach yoga on the sunbaked stones overlooking the glowing blue waters lapping the coastal town of Sliema at Exiles Beach Club. For a more luxurious experience, immerse yourself in the holistic Sanya Clinic in Naxxar, where you can practice a variety of yoga classes and enjoy top-tier spa treatments in one visit.

"I like to offer a class on a small, private beach on the summer solstice," explained Jennifer. "You take a set of stairs to go down from the road, and when you get there, you see a beach that's shaped like a semicircle. It's just you, looking toward the sun, at the sea, the sand, and the green grass. You don't see cars and roads, just this. On the solstice, the sun sets exactly in the middle of the beach. On that day, about a hundred of us gather here to offer sun salutations, set intentions, and kind of cleanse the past and make space for the future. This is for everyone, all levels. It's a great time of alignment, and you can feel very supported. We do a winter workshop as well. And then we also have full moon and new moon meditations during the week whenever they are. "That is the yoga scene here—it's very in tune with the rhythm of the world."

Visitors who come to savor Malta's connections with history should be sure not to miss out seeing the popular capital of Mdina, a walled fortress of a city that sits atop a hill, showcasing an eclectic mix of medieval and baroque stone architecture between charming narrow streets. "We have some fun foods, as well," noted Jennifer. "Be sure to get a Maltese pastizzi, with ricotta and peas. And to drink, there is the coffee shop, Sirkin, that's over a hundred years old. They put tea in a glass cup with a teaspoon, and they spend a full minute stirring the sugar into it. They keep up the tradition." Beyond historical cuisine, water-lovers might enjoy taking a ferry ride from Malta's mainland to the little island of Gozo, known for its laid-back vibe and snorkel-friendly beaches. On the even tinier island of Comino, the famous "crystal lagoon" will take your breath away with its astounding blue depths. Beyond the sea, check out the famous Bahrija trek, starting on the west side of Rabat, which meanders pleasantly past farmhouses built in the cliffside, old Roman excavations, and, in spring, meadows with more than a thousand species of plants bursting into flower. "My favorite little walk is to the Dingli cliffs," reflected Jennifer. "It's a secluded place to be on your own, to watch the sunset with literally no one around you but the rocks, the water, and the sun."

JENNIFER CORTIS, C.H.Ed (Dip Yoga), is a registered teacher with Yoga Alliance Professionals. She began practicing more than seventeen years ago and has pursued official yoga training with various yoga institutions. She has continued to take regular workshops throughout her teaching career, including yoga, meditation and tantra with Ananda Marga; yoga and anatomy and physiology at the Kevala Centre, UK; prana vinyasa flow with Shiva Rea at the Exhale Center for Sacred Movement, Venice, Los Angeles; Ayurveda with Maria Garre; bhakti yoga with Sri Chaitanya Saraswat Math; and vinyasa in the Krishnamacharya tradition with Mark Whitwell. In 2016, she was awarded the membership level of senior yoga teacher (SYT) with Yoga Alliance Professionals, which allows her to share her experience through Yoga Alliance CPD workshops in Malta for the continuing professional development of yoga teachers, advanced yoga practitioners, and health professionals. Her studio, Lotus Room, is based in Malta, and she hosts workshops there and in various places around Europe.

If You Go

▶ **Getting There**: Malta's airport, served by Air Malta (866-668-4820; airmalta.com), connects to most major European, North African, and Middle Eastern cities; travelers coming directly from the United States will likely need to connect in Paris or Rome.
▶ **Best Time to Visit**: Malta is sunny three-quarters of the year, but spring and early summer will spare you from the strongest heat.
▶ **Accommodations**: The Malta Tourism Authority (visitmalta.com) has a list of options, from luxe hotels to hostels to farm stays.

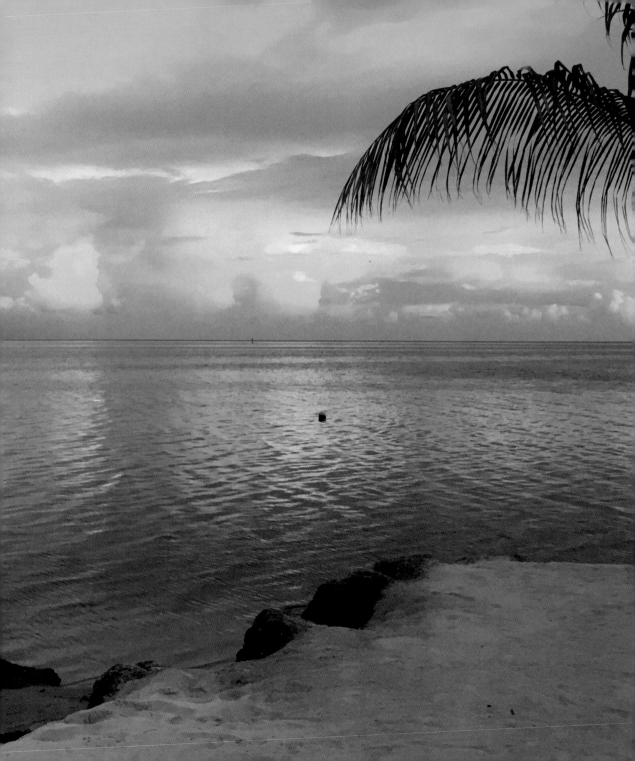

ISLAMORADA

RECOMMENDED BY **Lauren Ferrante**

A slice of island paradise that curves 120 miles into the Gulf of Mexico, the Florida Keys are not known for their abundance of shalas and ashrams. However, for yogis in the know, the Keys' lush climate, pockets of extreme solitude, and intimacy with the natural world all translate to a beautiful place to practice yoga—especially one you may have all to yourself.

"I moved here from Vermont in 2012," Lauren Ferrante began. "But when I arrived on Islamorada, I didn't find the yoga vibe I expected. Some people were teaching random classes here and there, but there was no real yoga presence on the island. So, I fast-tracked my plan, completed an intensive 200-plus-hours yoga teacher training in Mexico with a teacher out of Los Angeles, and started teaching the day after I got home. I wanted to tap into teaching within the natural beauty of the island. My 'studios' are absolutely incredible seaside locations surrounded by palm trees, water, sky, and sun."

There are technically more than sixteen islands in the string of the Keys, divided into six regions, each with its own personality, from raucous partyers to sport fishers and divers, to hammock-swinging vacationers. "Key Largo is the first island in the chain," Lauren explained. "You hit it after a seventeen-mile drive over the ocean from Miami, on a single stretch. It's very developed—it has Coral Reef State Park, so there's lots of scuba and snorkeling. But it's also very long, and it doesn't have as much nature as the other islands. Key West, which is the really big one, is at the very end of the chain. That's the busiest island, and it has more of a party vibe. Of course, it's beautiful; you can literally see Cuba on a clear day. But there's also lots of cruise ships and pub crawls. It's almost like a mini New Orleans. Islamorada, where Island Flow Yoga lives, is in the middle of the chain, and we're more like a village. It's a perfect mix of laid-back and slightly upscale, which is hard to explain because we're really not pretentious. There's classiness, but also a kind of fun Keys kitsch. We aren't

OPPOSITE:
The dreamy locale
of Islamorada
makes it
popular among
sport fishers
and yogis who
can't get enough
of the water.

a party island. We have some beautiful resorts and a few restaurants, but we're small, really small. Many people who live here are writers, shop owners, musicians, artists. It has a perfect small-town vibe and a strong community."

Islamorada, viewed from a map, is a razor-thin strip of land floating in the Atlantic; on the ground it's only 150 feet wide in some spots. Unsurprisingly, the community is oriented around the aquamarine ocean that surrounds the island, and water sports are plentiful, from parasailing, paddleboarding, and boating to deep-water snorkeling and diving. The island is also known to many as the sports fishing capital of the world, one of the places where saltwater fly-fishing was pioneered. Even if you don't have a favorite water sport, the opportunity to commune so intimately with the ocean has a profound effect. "One of my favorite things to do is be out on the water for sunset," reflected Lauren. "The colors reflect off the water and the sky and it's just . . . the word I want to use is 'god.' You feel a real connection to the Divine; the holy-s***-ness you look for when you travel stares you in the face every morning and every evening. It's beautiful and amazing and different every single day. It absolutely never gets old.

"My classes take place regardless of the weather. If we can't be on the beach, we are on decks or under open-air gazebos that extend into the water, so students are practicing right over the ocean or the bay," described Lauren. "But no matter where you practice on the island, when you're outside, you just get this incredible connection to nature. You'll look up during your practice and see a bird soaring above you, the clouds moving, the palm fronds blowing in a certain way, the sound of the water, the reflection of the light; it's a sensory experience. It's this connection to the living world that you can't get in a studio, and it's so nourishing.

"I was offering a sunset yoga event on a finger pier that goes out onto the bay. As we were practicing, a perfect double rainbow formed, a pod of dolphins appeared, and the sky was aglow. It was one of those perfect moments. Most everyone had tears streaming down their faces for the beauty of that experience. There is vulnerability and openness that can be accessed through the yoga practice. To be in that place and have the universe offer you the magic of connection to the natural world like that is profound. You can only have that moment once, but these moments are *all over* Islamorada. Yoga allows you to be present to them."

In 2017, misfortune struck the Keys in the form of Hurricane Irma. In the wake of the devastating storm surge and wind damage, hotels closed, homes were lost, and the tourism industry that fueled the island economy flatlined. But today, Islamorada has resurfaced as a community stronger than ever, with shops and beaches joyfully reopened, most hotels back at full speed, and the animal and plant life all but fully recovered.

"A beautiful thing is that we get people visiting Islamorada from all over the world," concluded Lauren. "They come here and practice with me in nature and they say, 'How can I ever go back to the walls of a studio after this?' I am so grateful that this is what I get to do every day."

LAUREN FERRANTE grew up in Long Beach, New York, and spent her days outdoors, running and biking along the beachside stretches. She went on to receive a master's degree in health and physical education with a minor in psychology. Yoga came into her life in 2002 when she moved to the Green Mountains of Vermont. In 2012, Lauren moved to the Florida Keys, where she felt compelled to share the benefits of yoga. She was presented an opportunity to give others a tool to deal with their own challenges, and she decided to follow her calling. After completing her 200-hour yoga teacher training in Mexico, she returned to the Keys and founded her business, Island Flow Yoga. Her insightful, intuitive, and down-to-earth vinyasa flow classes are held outdoors at some of the most stunning seaside locations in the Florida Keys. Lauren offers group classes, private sessions, yoga for your destination wedding, and other special events.

If You Go

▶ **Getting There**: The closest airport to Islamorada is in Miami, which is served by most major carriers. From there, it's an hour and a half drive.

▶ **Best Time to Visit**: The Florida Keys tend to be crowded December through March, and September marks the rainy season . . . but Islamorada is mostly sunny and warm year-round.

▶ **Accommodations**: Islamorada is home to several hotels, a favorite being Casa Morada, with its long pier stretching into the ocean (305-664-0044; casamorada.com). A helpful list of lodgings is available from the Islamorada Chamber of Commerce (islamorada chamber.com).

DESTINATION 22

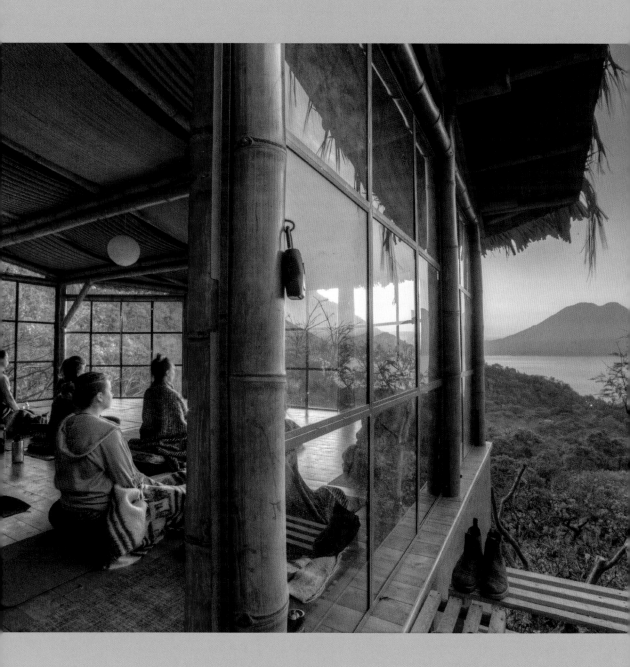

LAKE ATITLÁN

RECOMMENDED BY **Ali Dachis**

At one point in his travels, the English writer Aldous Huxley wrote that Lake Como, in northern Italy, was the "limit of the permissibly picturesque." When he later visited Lake Atitlán in the Guatemalan Highlands, Huxley described it as "Como with additional embellishments of several immense volcanoes."

Or just the *right* amount of a good thing for a yoga retreat.

"Yoga for me is about finding space, and a connection that's beyond your own comfort zone," Ali Dachis observed. "Coming to Guatemala was a step outside of my comfort zone. The Yoga Forest was recommended by a yoga-loving friend as an extraordinary place. The setting is very special—on the side of a mountain, overlooking Lake Atitlán. Different teachers cycle through, and the resort houses yoga teachers for free. In exchange, guest teachers do morning and afternoon classes. You're not sure what yoga you'll get as it depends on who's there."

Due to the civil war that tore the country on and off for nearly fifty years, Guatemala has not attracted as much tourist interest as neighboring Belize and Mexico's Yucatán Peninsula. Yet the small nation has much to offer, including nineteen different ecosystems (from mangrove swamps to lowland jungles to high woodlands), rich Mayan ruin sites, active volcanoes, tremendous diversity of bird life, and a friendly citizenry that warmly embraces visitors. (A peace accord was struck between warring factions in 1998, making travel more feasible for those uninterested in ducking the occasional insurgent bullet.) The Highlands region in the southern part of the country is especially dramatic, with Lake Atitlán the gem of the Sierra Madre. The lake—a caldera created by a volcanic eruption and filled by water—reaches depths of over a thousand feet and is flanked by three volcanoes to the south: San Pedro, Toliman, and Atitlán. The Mayan people believed

OPPOSITE:
Guests practice at
the Yoga Forest,
which overlooks
Lake Atitlán in
the Guatemalan
Highlands.

DESTINATION 23

its waters had healing qualities. In more recent times, many other spiritual seekers have been drawn here. (Some view Lake Atitlán as one of the world's energy vortexes.) It's possible to meet with local shamans, attend an Ayahuasca-fueled retreat, or expand your horizons through yoga at the Yoga Forest, which sits in a valley above the village of San Marcos La Laguna.

According to its website, the Yoga Forest was established as "a conscious living experiment, through a desire for living simply, greenly, and in communion with everything surrounding us." The concept here, where simple cabins and shalas mingle with ancient Mayan altars and natural springs, is "Deep Green Yoga," in which permaculture and a variety of wellness disciplines combine so that "the inherent wisdom of the entire ecosystem can fully flow, creating an open and thriving container for life and all expression." A lofty ambition, perhaps. But many Yoga Forest visitors seem to come away transformed, or, in the very least, deeply satisfied with their stay.

The special nature of a Yoga Forest visit is evident before you even set foot on the property. "It can be a complicated journey," Ali continued. "From Antigua, which is a tourist hub, it's a two-hour taxi ride to the lake. Then you board a boat for a short ride to San Marcos. From there, it's a thirty-minute hike up the mountain to the property. There are some signs, but I quickly became lost. Luckily, two local boys helped me get unlost." Comfortable rooms and sumptuous views of the lushly forested hillsides, Lake Atitlán, and the distant volcanoes are waiting once you reach the Yoga Forest, along with an opportunity to enhance your yoga practice.

"The classes are set up so anyone who's staying at the center and wants to attend can, but participation isn't mandatory," Ali said. "Sunrise yoga is a simple vinyasa practice. The afternoon session is more vigorous. The shala overlooks the lake, and the views are stunningly beautiful. You can take in both the sunrise and the sunset. Overall, I found the yoga sessions easeful, but more challenging in a spiritual way than my practice at home. I found it useful to approach things with a beginner's brain, to go back to basics in a way I might not seek day-to-day. After all, things are a lot slower on the side of a mountain in Guatemala." Although the styles of practice available will vary depending on which teachers are in residence, guests can generally count on teaching and practice in jnana yoga, raja/ashtanga yoga, bhakti yoga, and karma yoga.

As part of its permaculture philosophy, all the vegetarian food served at the Yoga Forest is organically grown on the hillsides by farmers employed by the retreat.

(Composting toilets help complete the circle.) "Many meals consist of rice and beans with a variety of spices, plus veggies, and are delicious," Ali described. "They are a community experience; everyone joins to help out. There are opportunities to volunteer to work with the farmers if you wish." There are ample opportunities to explore the area through hikes or forays to the lake. "Some people visit San Marcos La Laguna, where you can shop and get energy work," Ali added. "But I stayed on the side of the mountain. It's just too beautiful, and all of your needs are taken care of." (Guests are asked to store phones and other electronics in the Yoga Forest office, where they can be used only when you have to be in touch with family.)

Incredible vistas, a deeply spiritual setting, and an eclectic assembly of instructors can all contribute to a memorable yoga retreat. Ali was also taken with the kind of people who chose to visit a place like the Yoga Forest. "The conversations during and after dinner were mind-opening," she offered. These were curious people, seeking some kind of connection. I remember thinking that I didn't know people could make the choices they did—volunteering at Yoga Forest for a year, traveling full-time. These were some of the most eye-opening conversations I've had."

ALI DACHIS began her yoga journey studying ashtanga, and began practicing vinyasa and other styles shortly after. She fell in love with the movement and mindfulness of yoga, and found that it opened her eyes to the stability and beauty in life. Ali is certified to teach vinyasa yoga by CorePower Yoga, and laughter yoga. She is always excited to spread the amazing power of yoga to all who seek unity in life, on and off the mat. In her classes, Ali shares the sense of community, strength, and peace she has found through the practice of yoga, and currently calls New York City home.

If You Go

▶ **Getting There**: Most visitors fly into Guatemala City, which is in the Highlands region and is served by many major carriers, including American (800-433-7300; aa.com), Continental (800-523-3273; continental.com), and Delta (800-221-1212; delta.com). From the airport, it's roughly an hour shuttle to Antigua, where you'll overnight. From

Antigua, it's a roughly four-hour shuttle to San Marcos La Laguna, or you can take a shuttle to San Pedro and a boat the rest of the way to San Marcos. It's a forty-minute hike to the Yoga Forest.

▶ **Best Time to Visit**: Retreats and classes are offered at the Yoga Forest throughout the year. November through May is drier and warmer; April through October sees cooler temperatures and afternoon showers. August and September—hurricane season—has potential for the heaviest rain.

▶ **Accommodations**: The Yoga Forest (502 33011835; theyogaforest.org) offers comfortable rooming options, farm-to-table vegetarian fare, and a variety of themed retreats and trainings.

KAPAAU

RECOMMENDED BY **Amanda Webster**

America's rainbow state, the Hawaiian Islands are famed for their balmy blue oceans, intoxicating flowers, and lush greenery at every turn. Such a soothing place is no stranger to yoga, but it's also not always the island paradise you would expect. "The Big Island," or Hawaii Island, has the most environmental variety of any of its sister islands. The western side consists of a dry, sunny, California-like climate that draws most of the tourist traffic. However, on the island's eastern side, the capital city, Hilo, is surrounded by dewy rainforest and moves at a slower pace, giving you more of a sense for how year-round residents of the island live. In the middle of the island are the coffee plantations (Kona Coffee Living History Farm offers yoga classes among the precious greenery) and the weird, moon-like landscape of the volcanoes Mauna Kea and Mauna Loa. And then there's the active lava field of Kilauea on the southeastern side, a primordial planet of ominous black waves and oozing lava. For yogis looking for a more luxurious but still intimately and authentically Hawaiian experience, the Hawaii Island Retreat Center beckons.

"Hawaii is home to me, and I wanted to do something at home," began Amanda Webster. "There's so much history and culture and outdoor activity in Hawaii. Yoga is popular, of course. I had been hosting yoga retreats at rental houses, but that wasn't sustainable or something I wanted to do long term. Then the Hawaii Island Retreat Center presented itself. It is one of the only retreat centers in Hawaii that was sustainable, designed for group gatherings, and not camping oriented. It was perfect."

Set at the top of a large emerald hill overlooking the sea, the center rolls outward in a tiered expanse of white columns, with a vast, mirror-surfaced infinity pool at the doorstep reflecting the sky. "The original owner was inspired by King Kamehameha, who liked classical Italian architecture," Amanda noted. "Beyond the entryway, a ylang ylang tree

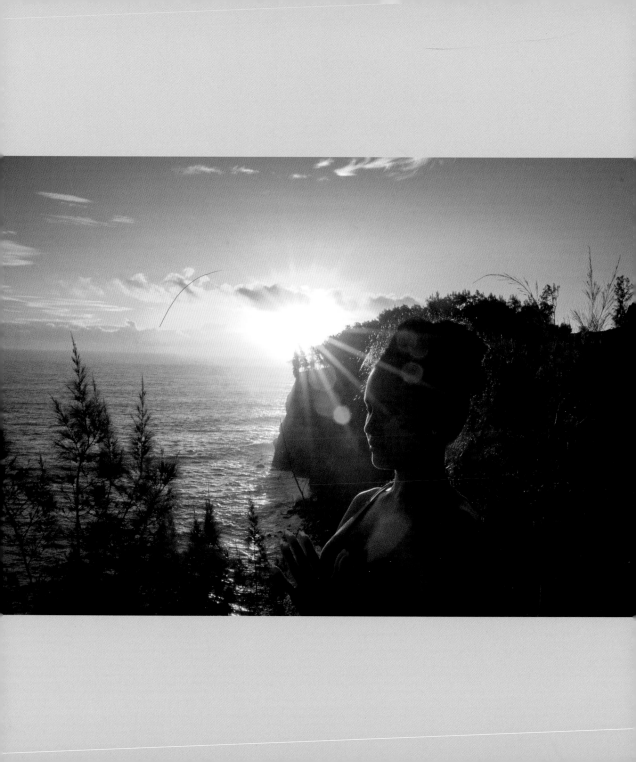

grows in the center courtyard, and the scent of the flowers floats down every hall. There are hotel rooms and bungalows, and yurts up on the hill. The whole place is bordered by the valley and the ocean. There are pine trees, meadows, and gardens where the owners grow food to feed guests. There are chickens and goats too. It's a bounty. It's beautiful."

Hawaii Island Retreat Center rests at Ahu Pohaku Ho'omaluhia, which translates to "The Gathering Place of Peace-giving Stones," in the town of Kapaau. The two-story eco-boutique is intimate yet expansive, with twenty rooms situated on fifty-five acres. The outdoor spa pavilion hosts the very best of Hawaii's massage therapists, healers, cultural experts, and outdoor guides. Amanda noted, "It is believed that King Kamehameha used to have his royal councils here. The feel is something you need to experience yourself. There's something really intangible about this place."

"The very first time I stayed there, we were sleeping in a yurt," Amanda recalled. "I woke up in the middle of the night and heard chanting. It scared me a little because there was nothing nearby, no community centers, no other hotels. The center is all by itself. So, we asked the owner the next day who was chanting, and she said that there was no event. It was just the land welcoming us. I know it can sound hard to believe, but this truly moved me. There really is something special about this place."

A weeklong retreat at the center allows yogis to immerse themselves in Hawaii's natural wonders, inviting spiritual contemplation in tune with its history and landscape. "This whole place is a full sensory experience," Amanda described. "There's a hardwood floor studio, with sliding doors that open onto the ocean view, where yoga and meditation are typically practiced. We tend to forgo music, because you can hear the ocean and the pine trees moving. Above the center, there's a little hill overlooking the ocean, and you can go sit right on the ledge, practically in the sky. Or you can go over by the reading room and sit among the treetops and hear the birds chirping. There's a mile or two of gentle trails that cover the grounds, so you can walk freely among all of this. You can visit the farm and the animals. I always encourage people to come for two extra days because there's so much to do."

For those wishing to explore beyond the center, a vast array of experiences await, from touring Hawaii's prolific, rolling farmland, to snorkeling among the fish in the island's brilliant blue waters. "You can go ziplining through the forest," Amanda continued. "There's an immense number of hiking trails. You can also go fluming (which is a bit like floating in a tube on a river) in old sugar plantation canals, with a tour of the history as

DESTINATION

OPPOSITE:
Sunset on
the island of
Hawaii offers a
brilliant moment
for gratitude
and reflection.

you go. Or you can go even farther into the island and check out the city of Hilo, or all the riches at Hawai'i Volcanoes National Park. On our retreats, I generally like to take a group to Mauna Kea for stargazing. There's something for everyone, depending on how active and outdoorsy you want to be."

Given the number of tourists that flock here, many Hawaiians have become concerned with preserving the island chain's natural beauty. To do its part, the Hawaiian Island Retreat Center boasts trend-setting eco-spa practices, designed for harmony and balance with nature. "They're sustainable," Amanda explained. "They employ water catchment and solar and wind power. They grow the vast majority of food we eat in the garden. It's important to us to keep in step with sustainability culture as a whole, a nod to the past and the future. There's a big movement on Hawaii to go back to the way things used to be and live off the grid. It draws on a lot of classic practices that have a real practicality. There's a fusion of past/present in Hawaii that's really represented at this place."

Whether it is meditation over the ocean, sunbathing on black-sand beaches, or savoring homegrown meals, paradisiacal Hawaii is notorious for melting even the most skeptical hearts. "Even people who don't do yoga or meditation come here with their spouses or friends, and often at the end of their stay, they've had some sort of profound or important insight," Amanda ventured. "You can feel grounded even if the thing you're getting clarity on is uncomfortable. There's something here that allows you to feel settled."

AMANDA WEBSTER is an eRYT-500 certified yoga teacher and founder of Amanda Webster Wellness based on the Big Island of Hawaii. She holds a master's degree in psychology and is a certified Ayurveda counselor through the American Institute of Vedic Studies, often incorporating the holistic practices of Ayurveda into her teaching. Amanda loves Hawaii's dynamic contrasting landscapes—from desert to snow and from ocean to lush rainforest—and its healing energy. She has an intuitive, down-to-earth approach to teaching, practicing, counseling, and embodying yoga through her lifestyle. She is known for her ability to establish a strong community, inspiring connection, sustainability, and self-inquiry through a wide variety of high-quality yoga classes, trainings, and retreats on the Big Island and the mainland.

▶ **Getting There**: You can fly into either smaller Hilo International Airport on the island's eastern side, or much larger Kona International Airport on the western side. Both are served by Hawaiian Airlines (877-426-4537; hawaiianairlines.com) and Southwest Airlines (800-435-9792; southwest.com)

▶ **Best Time to Visit**: The winter months are generally rainiest, but the tropical island sees some showers any time of year. Spring and fall see fewer tourist crowds.

▶ **Accommodations**: Hawaii Island Retreat Center is bookable at hawaiiislandretreat.com, with more hotel options available at the Hawaii Tourism Board at gohawaii.com.

24

DESTINATION

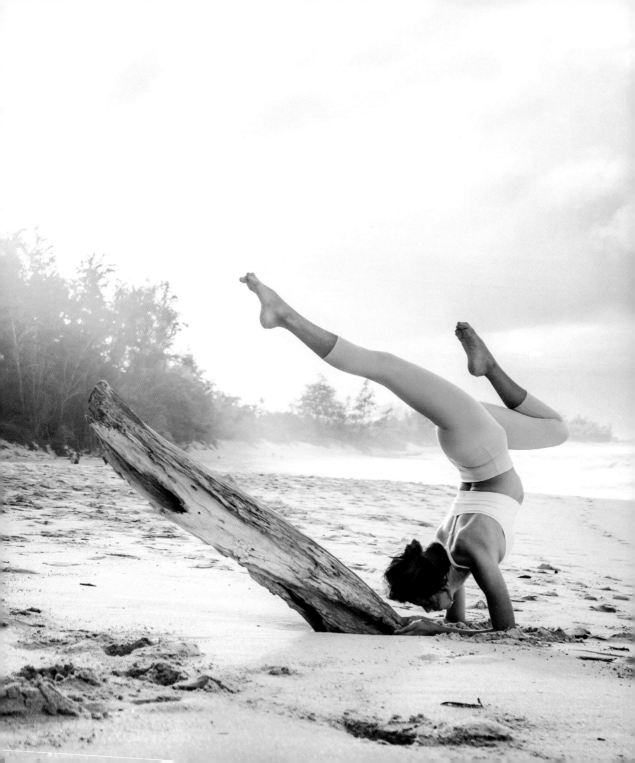

MAUI

RECOMMENDED BY **Jennifer Lynn**

The Hawaiian Islands are the crown jewel of the Northern Pacific, with each island in the chain holding a distinct personality. Oahu is famous for its upscale shopping and family friendliness. Hawaii, "The Big Island," boasts acres of eerie lava and a population of mild-mannered scientists and farmers. Then there's Maui, the second-largest island in the chain, known for its vast hiking trails, tranquil towns, and all-around chill, hippie vibe. This is the island where time slows down.

"When I first got off the plane here, I felt my knees almost buckle," reflected Jennifer Lynn. "Listen, I'm a logical person—a mathematician—and we math-heads are usually logical, but as I was standing on the tarmac, seeing the West Maui Mountains in front of me and Haleakala behind me, I felt like I was supposed to drop to my knees and bow."

The "Valley Isle," as it's often called, is mostly two hundred feet below sea level, except for its east and west ends, which surge into the sky as the West Maui Mountains to the west and the sky-shattering Haleakala in the east. Along the northeastern shore runs the famous Road to Hana, a winding freeway, passing through fragrant green jungle, secluded beaches, iridescent waterfalls, and stunning bluffs overlooking the Pacific. From the bamboo forest hike, the mana-charging glory of Iao Valley, the thundering Seven Sisters waterfalls, and the many miles of swimmable coastline (more than any of its sister islands), Maui is a nature-lover's paradise.

Although it hosts only about twenty regular yoga studios in its seven hundred square miles, the opportunity to connect with the elements is what has made this island famous among yogis. (Famed ashtanga master Nancy Gilgoff has her home studio here, although the address is kept secret.) All the studios seek to connect the practitioners to yogic roots in harmony with the nature around them.

OPPOSITE:

The philosophies of yoga blend brilliantly with Maui's divine beauty.

DESTINATION

25

"There are so many wonderful studios in Maui," continued Jennifer, "so many ways to work with nature. In ours, we wanted to honor the flow of creation. The name 'Wisdom Flow' came to me walking in the forest one day. Everywhere in the world, there is a sense of life as a flow, but it is really apparent in Maui. So, in the central part of the studio we have a big mural, a tree murti and tree devi—the three gods and goddesses paired up. It begins with Brahma, representing inception and new beginnings, and his consort Saraswati, who is a reminder to think before beginning something and make sure whatever you're doing is aligned with you and the environment around you. Then you have Vishnu and Lakshmi. Vishnu is the god of respect, maintenance, appreciation. He's often called the great main-tainer, reminding us to love what we've built, to care for it, show up for it, clean it, so that it can continue to serve us. And Lakshmi, his consort, reminds us to say, 'I love it, I love that energy. I am here to celebrate that with my gold coins.' And then Shiva and Durga are there to represent the liberating current, the reminder that everything that we create, every relation-ship, must have a day of transition where it begins to shed its form and dissolve back into pure energy. Durga is the quintessential mother saying, 'Don't worry about the sh** hitting the fan. Go ahead and let go. Surrender. We will pick things up and make them better.' So, this is all in a wave in the center of the studio, a reminder of the flow of the universe, the flow of nature."

The intimate connections with nature and community that Maui is so famous for continue as you step out of the studio. The annual Butterfly Effect Festival, a community of noncompetitive women's watersports festival produced by Tatiana Howard, began here in 2007 before spreading across the world. The event still takes place on Baldwin Beach every year, with a free yoga class. In the town of Makena, the community-based Quepasana retreat center offers guests seven-day Vipassana silent retreats, supported with food and massage right on the ocean—for free. "It's a nonprofit dedicated to helping people awak-en to their own heart," described Jennifer.

"There's also a spa called Hale Ho'omana, which translates to 'house of empowerment.' It's on the mountain, run by a magical Hawaiian woman named Gina Nalawi; she is a sor-ceress, a goddess. This is not your normal beauty spa experience. She has created, very intentionally, a sacred space there, with gardens and herbs and waterways. She makes some of the healing potions and oils that native Hawaiians made hundreds of years ago. She's cultivating and preserving her culture in a beautiful way.

"That's the thing about Maui. It's unbelievable," concluded Jennifer. "The beauty and glory of source energy—what we sometimes call god—is just *in your face* here. You can't get away from it. There's no turning it off or shutting it out. The mountains speak to you. The vastness of the ocean, representing infinite expansion and boundless possibility, is always in view. And the community has put in place special, thoughtful county laws to preserve this bounty. For example, there are laws on how many lights you can build, to ensure that everyone can see the stars shine, and limits on the size of large freeways so they don't inhibit the nature around them. Everything is built to preserve the island's beauty. And when you're interacting with that beauty every day, it makes it easier when you tap into your asana practice to find the divine."

JENNIFER LYNN holds a BA in math and computer science from San Jose State University and worked as an engineer for Hewlett-Packard before coming home to yoga after a battle with cancer. Jennifer spent eight years training and researching to find the heart of yoga so she could offer it with purity and clarity to her students. On a yoga retreat in Maui twenty years ago, Jennifer felt the call of the island and left her old life in California to begin again. After teaching at a few different studios on the island, she is now the owner and director of Wisdom Flow Yoga School on Maui, offering ongoing classes and teacher training programs based on aligning body and mind to allow our natural well-being and joy to flow through us.

DESTINATION

25

If You Go

▶ **Getting There**: Kahului Airport is a hub of Hawaiian Airlines (877-426-4537; hawaiian airlines.com), but Alaska Airlines also offers several flights (800-654-5669; alaskaair.com).
▶ **Best Time to Visit**: Maui has a tropical climate, with warm days and showers year-round, with a bit more rainy days in winter and early spring. Some insiders say early fall is the best balance between crowds and rain clouds.
▶ **Accommodations**: Maui offers everything from luxurious five-star hotels in Lahaina such as the Montage Kapalua Bay (808-662-6600; montagehotels.com/kapaluabay), to camping by the beach, such as at Waianapanapa State Park (808-984-8109; dlnr.hawaii.gov). The Hawaiian Tourism Authority offers a range of accommodations at gohawaii.com.

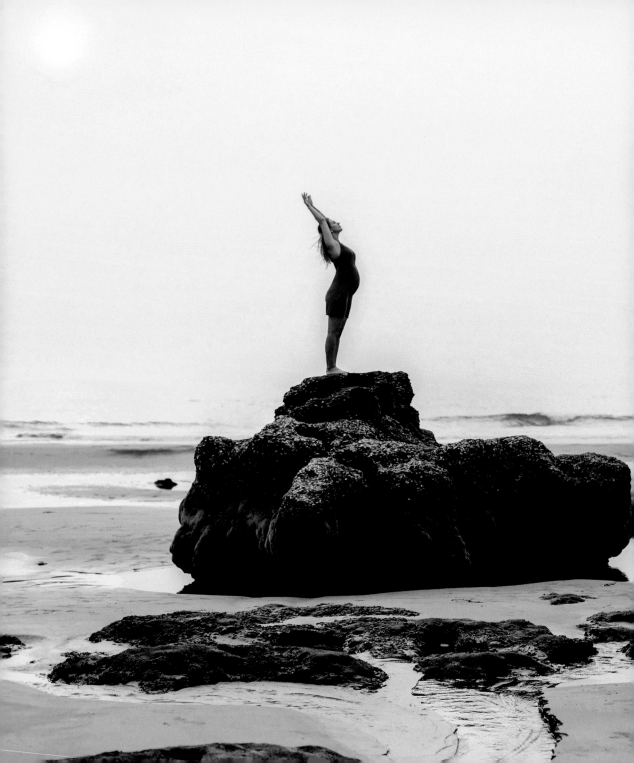

India

GOA

RECOMMENDED BY **Lalita Marmeka**

For those wishing to connect to the motherland of yoga but who also are seeking the serenity of a beach town, the leisurely, laid-back coastal state of Goa awaits. "You can't run anywhere in Goa without seeing a yoga center," began Lalita Marmak. "I always say to people who've never been to India that Goa is a really nice landing spot. It's such a vibrant, bustling, raw place. Goa is probably India's most liberal area, at least on the coast, and the most used to having tourists. It's more acceptable for women to be in bikinis, for example, rather than covered as you might have to be in other states. A lot of hippies came in the sixties and seventies and never left. It's always been quite a hub for yoga."

Goa, located on the western edge of the Indian coast, has long been a respite for the citizens of nearby mega-metropolises like Mumbai, Delhi, and Bangalore, looking to escape the smog and bustle of the city in exchange for crystal clear water, soft sand, and swaying palm trees. Although yoga shalas here have been welcoming Western hippies since the 1960s, the region's history with Europeans actually dates back centuries before that. In the early 1500s, the Catholic Portuguese colonized the area, kicking out the Adil Shahi dynasty that reigned over most of South India at the time. The Portuguese colonists stayed for hundreds of years until Goa became part of India in 1961 (fourteen years after the rest of the country claimed independence from Britain). The Catholic influences of Portuguese rule have left their mark on Goa, with numerous European colonial buildings and Iberian-style churches spread throughout the region. However, the vibe in Goa does not inherit much strictness from either of its former Catholic or Muslim overlords. Instead, it is often described by locals as *susegaad*, a word derived from Portuguese and Konkani (the official language of the State of Goa) that refers to a luxurious, easygoing way of life.

OPPOSITE:
Influenced by
the cultures of
ancient India
and Portugal,
Goa has been
welcoming
foreign yogis
and Indian
vacationers
for decades.

DESTINATION **26**

In North Goa's upscale Mandrem district, quiet streets, candy-colored beach bungalows, tucked-away cafés, and yoga retreats abound. Mandrem is also the home of one of the first yoga centers founded in Goa: Ashiyana—a tropical cluster of wooden staircases, Rajasthani-decorated suites, thatched-roof huts, beachwood bridges, and open-air shalas, sheltered in the jungle between the Mandrem beach and river.

"*Ashiyana* means 'home' in Hindi, and that's how I felt the first time I came here—like I had found my home," reflected Lalita. "There is this iconic wooden bridge over the river that you cross to get to the main center, and the trees hanging over it have heart-shaped leaves. The first time I walked across the bridge, one of these leaves fell and landed right on my feet. I have had so many profound moments on this bridge.

"The center has five yoga shalas," Lalita continued. "The main one is a big, open, wooden shala, where I taught my first official class after completing teacher training. It's raised two steps off the ground and has coconut palm trees growing up through it. It's a very natural, healing, and sacred place. You can practice and see the gardens, which are so beautiful, so luscious and green.

"Across the bridge from the center is Mandrem beach, which is what most people know us for. "It's vast and secluded, and the sea is shallow for quite far out as well. It doesn't have the white sand some people look for, but it's beautiful in its own way. Surfing lessons have started recently, but mostly it's people walking, sitting in the beach huts in the sand dunes, lounging, enjoying everything.

"Because we are living among nature, it's best if you like animals if you come to Goa," noted Lalita. "We have squirrels, frogs, grasshoppers, birds, crabs—nothing scary, but there's a lot of activity. Ashiyana 'has' four rescue dogs that pop in and out of classes from time to time. Dogs are our best teachers, I think," Lalita said with a laugh. "Savasana is their favorite pose—they are all masters of it."

No Goa visit would be complete without a brief trip eastward from the beach to explore the treasures of the region's interior. Tour spice plantations and observe sacred plants in their natural environment, buy a ticket to a "tiatir" show (Goa's famous Broadway-style plays, often on political themes), or browse the "hippie flea markets" in Anjuna, where Tibetan sculptures, Kerala spices, and Rajasthani bedspreads mingle with bongs, Levi's, and T-shirts for one of the most colorful shopping experiences in India. The Dudhsagar waterfall walk, a short day trip from Mandrem, takes visitors past a series of breathtakingly tall waterfalls, thundering through the jungle.

DESTINATION

26

One of the special aspects of Ashiyana is the sense of intimacy the center exudes. "A lot of the local members of staff are related," Lalita added. "It's very relaxed, a really homey vibe. You're enveloped in a loving embrace as soon as you arrive. We have a lot of solo travelers, but they don't stay solo for long—they make lifelong friends. Very often people will come here and then come back again here at the same time every year. Goa is a family."

LALITA MARMEKA first discovered yoga as a necessary medicine during a challenging chapter of her life. Inspired by the healing benefits she experienced from her own practice, her interests in a more conscious existence led her to India, completing her two-hundred-hour yoga teacher training at Ashiyana Goa in 2012. As well as offering yoga and bodywork, she created the hugely popular "Ecstatic Shaking" drop-in sessions that she has held at Ashiyana Goa since 2015. In 2017, Lalita spent a life-changing four weeks in Bali, training to facilitate 5Elements Dance Activation™ Journeys with Malaika MaVeena Darville. This experience further stoked her passion for dance, breath, movement, connection, and play. When not in India, Lalita can be found shaking her way around London, Ibiza, and the British countryside.

DESTINATION

26

If You Go

▶ **Getting There**: Visitors can fly directly into Goa via Dabolim airport, served by carriers including IndiGo (+91 1246173838; goindigo.in) and SpiceJet (+91 9871803333; spicejet.com), but most international flights will land in nearby Mumbai. From there, you can take a train or an overnight bus to the coast.

▶ **Best Time to Visit**: The best time of the year to visit Goa is mid-November to mid-February, when the weather is comfortable, dry, and pleasant. Winds often pick up in May and June.

▶ **Accommodations**: Ashiyana Goa (+91 9850401714; ashiyana.com) is one of the oldest yoga retreat centers in Goa. A variety of hotels and ashrams are also bookable online ahead of time at goa-tourism.com.

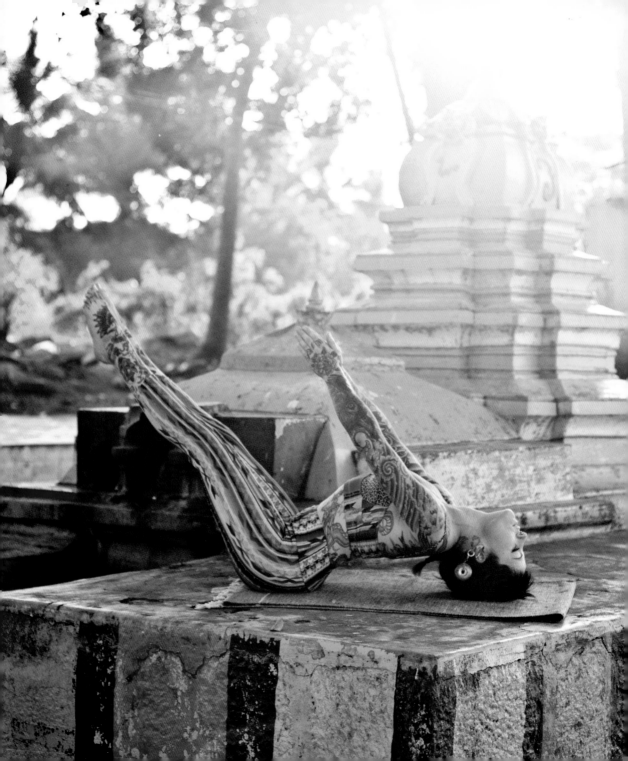

MYSURU (MYSORE)

RECOMMENDED BY **Didi von Deck**

The Ashtanga Yoga Research Institute was founded in Mysuru, India, by K. Pattabhi Jois in 1948. Since then, the physically demanding, fixed-sequence style has been spreading across the globe like wildfire, especially embraced by Western culture. Over the past thirty years, although it has remained a fixed discipline, ashtanga has been source material for vinyasa flow styles, power yoga, and the everyday "yoga-as-exercise" classes you now see regularly across the West. But most of that work started about seventy years ago in Mysuru.

"Krishnamacharya, who lived from 1888 to 1989, is considered the father of modern yoga," explained Didi von Deck. "He taught yoga to the maharaja of Mysuru and then started a yoga school at the palace. He taught yoga to the future founding teachers B. K. S. Iyengar and K. Pattabhi Jois, among others. So, Mysuru is famous for the Jois family's ashtanga studios, but Iyengar and other styles of yoga are taught there as well. Most people think Mysuru is just about ashtanga, but it's a bit more like Rishikesh; it's a city dedicated to yoga."

Many devout ashtangis will make the pilgrimage to Mysuru (known as Mysore until the government officially de-anglicized the name in 2014) to learn from the Jois family. "I went to Mysuru because I was curious about how this form of yoga came about," mused Didi. "I think anyone who does yoga for a long time and feels the effects starts to ask questions. And every time I asked my teachers questions about ashtanga, the conversation kept going back to Mysuru."

Although K. Pattabhi Jois passed from this world in 2009, Mysuru remains the face of the family's yoga institutions. His daughter Saraswathi teaches at the Shri K. Pattabhi Jois Ashtanga Yoga Institute (KPJAYI), and his grandson Sharath recently opened the Sharath Yoga Center nearby. Both offer certifications in the famous style that cannot be

OPPOSITE: Yoga weaves seamlessly into the bustling city of Mysuru, the home of ashtanga.

DESTINATION

27

127

obtained anywhere else. "It's true that it's hard to get in to work with the Jois family," explained Didi. "You have to apply online three months in advance, and Sharath's program fills in less than five minutes. There are many ashtanga teachers in Mysuru like B. K. S. Iyengar and others, where you can get a smaller student-to-teacher ratio and learn pranayama, philosophy, and meditation as well as the ashtanga sequences of poses. There are lots of different ways to practice."

Known as "the city of palaces," Mysuru has been a popular South Indian tourist destination for centuries and is considered the cultural capital of South Karnataka. Famous for its shopping markets, which feature premium silk saris (the city produces 70 percent of India's mulberry silk), sandalwood incense, essential oils, as well as its street food snacks like Mysuru pak (a chewy sweet made of roasted gram flour and ghee) and masala dosa (a thin pancake of fermented batter, topped with garlic chutney and spiced potatoes), most visiting yogis are happy that they are not restricted to staying inside at a center during their pilgrimage. Mysuru Palace, one of the seven palaces that grace the former set of India's Wadiyar dynasty, is recognized as the second most visited Indian tourist destination. With its red-domed tops, lush gardens, and meticulously preserved interiors, it's easy to see why more than six million people visit every year.

Mysuru is not only the home of ashtanga yoga, but also a center of general spiritual inquiry. It's home to India's first academic Ayurvedic medical institution (established in 1908) as well as Sanskrit scholars, traditional doctors, and massage therapists. Learned well-being is a way of life for the bustling city. "It's a cacophony," Didi continued. "Birds are calling constantly, and their songs mix with the cries of vendors walking the streets to hawk their wares. Festivals are celebrated with parades through the streets and people singing, chanting, and dancing. There are scooters and rickshaws and cows and goats and traffic and honking horns (but very few accidents!). It's hot and dusty. And so much brilliant color—the clothing, fruits, and flowers in the Devaraja Market, the garlands that adorn the statues of deities. It's still a city, though; sometimes you catch a whiff of sewage or rotting garbage, or pass through the slums dotted with fires for cooking and chickens scratching in the dirt, but then there's the scent of incense, wafting from a temple or a guard room. There are little temples everywhere."

Staying in a home is the most common way visiting yogis stay in Mysuru, as most centers are not ashrams in the traditional sense and don't offer overnight stays. However, this allows for a deeper appreciation and connection with Mysuru life. "People are really helpful and sincere," reflected Didi. "They think we're sort of funny, but they are willing to help you out. There are lots of little quirks to living in Mysuru. Electricity outages are common. Maybe there's a generator, but maybe not. Maybe the running water stops. You learn how to adapt.

"One thing my daughter noticed here is that the Divine—the spiritual—is woven into daily life. It's not like the West. You don't need to be religious to feel the spirituality. From the festivals to the parades, visiting the temples, just walking down the street, you realize that your life, the life of the gods, and the layers of existence are all one continuum, happening at the same time. It's all just right in front of you. It is so *accessible*."

DIDI VON DECK began learning ashtanga yoga three weeks after her third child was born. Despite the challenges of raising her family and pursuing her career as an orthopedic surgeon, she eventually started a daily practice under Kate O'Donnell and has since studied with David Swenson, Nancy Gilgoff, David Williams, and Richard Freeman. She travels to India frequently to study ashtanga yoga with the Jois family and was authorized to teach ashtanga by Saraswathi Jois. While in India, she continues her studies of Sanskrit, chanting, and yoga philosophy, and she takes time to work with the Odanadi Seva Trust, an organization that works to rescue, rehabilitate, reintegrate, and empower trafficked and sexually exploited women and children (Yoga Stops Traffick). Didi also teaches Feldenkrais Awareness Through Movement® and is the director of the Mysore ashtanga program at the Down Under School of Yoga in her hometown of Boston.

DESTINATION

27

If You Go

▶ **Getting There**: The nearest major airport to Mysuru is in Bangalore, about a hundred miles away. From here, Mysuru can be reached by bus, car, or train.

▶ **Best Time to Visit**: The best time to visit Mysuru is during the monsoon season and winter months, from July to February, with most rain concentrated in September and October. Temperatures are higher from March to May.

▶ **Accommodations**: Homestays are the most common for students studying at KPJAYI; these can be found on Facebook groups and at homestay.com.

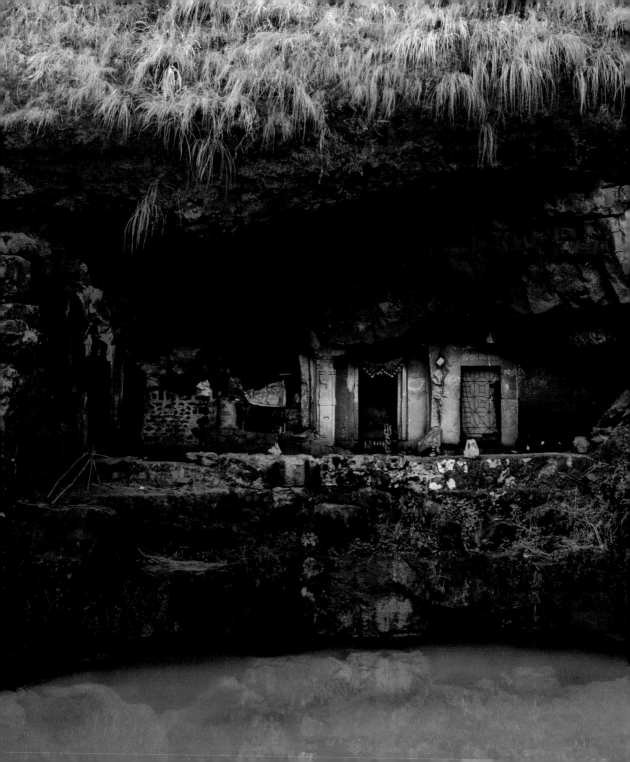

PUNE

RECOMMENDED BY **Lorenzo Sacchini**

"With every yoga tradition, there is a place, a city that is symbolic to that lineage, where the guru lived and has his institute," began Lorenzo Sacchini. "Pune is the home of Iyengar yoga. It is a place you really should try to go to, especially if you are a dedicated practitioner or teacher."

Pune, also known as "Poona," has spent the last few decades stepping out of the shadow of its more famous neighbor, Mumbai, and carving its own niche on the Indian map. Located in the center of the country, with a cool, breezy climate that encourages lush greenery and temperate summers, the city boasts a strong international community and position of prominence. This is due in part to its rich history as seat of the Peshwas (the prime ministers of the eighteenth-century Maratha Empire) and its gurus. Although most come to study at the Ramamani Iyengar Memorial Yoga Institute (RIMYI), the famous leader of the Rajneeshi's, Osho, once lived here, and his followers still keep an active ashram. "My impression when I got there was that it's quite intense," continued Lorenzo. "Compared to Mumbai, it's a country village, but it still has three million people in one city. On the one hand, everyone is everywhere doing everything. But at the same time there's this atmosphere of the sacred, of ancient practices, of respect. Somehow, they manage to have this many people together and it has this sacred feeling. When I first came, I think I imagined it would be in a quiet zone that's surrounded by nature, but RIMYI is actually just in the middle of a busy street in the suburbs. It feels just as powerful as if it was alone on a hill."

B. K. S. Iyengar (often affectionately referred to as "Guruji") originally founded his eponymous branch of yoga as a way to heal from tuberculosis. The style has a particular emphasis on props to accommodate a variety of body shapes and to encourage, above all,

OPPOSITE: Pune, the headquarters of Iyengar yoga, is a city rich in hidden alleys, secret spaces, and architectural wonders.

DESTINATION 28

proper alignment during postures. This proper physical alignment is said to be the gateway to alignment of the mind. Founded in 1976, RIMYI in Pune remains the mother institute of Iyengar yoga worldwide, a beacon for students and teachers across the globe. Prashant and Abhijata Iyengar (Guruji's son and granddaughter, respectively) continue to teach and evolve the method that is one of the world's most widely practiced yogas.

"Going to the institute charges you up like a battery and keeps you inspired," reflected Lorenzo. "It's really important as a teacher to have this reference. Ultimately, yoga was given to you. It's important to have this feedback and this relationship where you keep yourself updated and in line with the tradition. Being there also provides a wonderful opportunity to meet so many other practitioners from all over the world who are like you, but from literally everywhere."

Most yogis come to study at RIMYI for a month, under the structure of the prestigious teachers therein. Daily classes with rotating teachers, along with time for self-practice, are paired with opportunities for class observation, to see other teaching methods and student–teacher interactions. The institute offers a variety of children's classes, classes for seniors, and therapy classes to accommodate all different needs. For those looking for a place of deep commitment to their practice, this experience is unparalleled. "I was at the institute Monday to Saturday for six hours a day. You only have time to eat and sleep when you are not at the institute. You rent an apartment close by so that you can save most of your energy for being at the institute. Even my teacher said [not to spend too much energy exploring the city]."

This is good advice, as Pune is home to many treasures besides RIMYI. Trees and lush forests coexist with majestic buildings like the Aga Khan Palace, which served as a prison for Mahatma Gandhi during the Indian independence movement, and the 2,000-year-old Sinhagad Fort, covered in vines and myths of battles past. The famous Shaniwar Wada, the seat of India's Maratha Empire for most of the eighteenth century, attracts the most tourists. Beyond the historical riches, Pune is famous for its shopping and nightlife, with many international headliners booking concerts. There are a plethora of yogi-friendly eats as well, from high-end restaurants to street fare. You can even visit India's oldest Parsi bakery, Kayani, for a vegetarian treat.

However, if connection with Hindu treasures is more appealing than shopping or snacking, the green hills around Pune offer tremendous treasures. "I became friends with a rickshaw driver named Nana," reflected Lorenzo. "He would come around and drive us to different temples. Anyone who goes must visit the Pataleshwar caves—it's beautiful and so close to the institute. It's a temple dedicated to Shiva, carved into a single block of basalt rock thousands of years ago. You can also go to Parvati Hill, the oldest structure in Pune, a temple situated on top of a hillock, dedicated to the consort of Lord Shiva. From the top of the hill, you can look down and see the whole city."

"The first time I went, it was Ganesh Chaturthi, the birthday of Ganesh," remembered Lorenzo. "It's a festival that goes on for ten days. People build up these Ganesh statues and mini temples, and then, on the birthday, they march toward the river and immerse the idols. The main ceremony is huge. There are music, dancers, ceremonies—there's always some kind of ceremony in India. Whenever you go at any time of the year, you're always going to see a festival.

"It's really beautiful. I'm always sad when I have to come home from Pune."

LORENZO SACCHINI discovered Iyengar yoga in 2013, when he started practicing at the Central Yoga School in Australia, and has been passionate about it ever since. Now a certified junior intermediate Iyengar practitioner, he visits India yearly to further improve his teaching and understanding of the practice, occasionally contributing guest articles about his experience to various yoga blogs. He currently lives in Sydney, where he teaches classes at Central Yoga School.

If You Go

▶ **Getting There**: Lohegaon Airport is an international airport, served by most major carriers, especially AirAsia (airasia.com), Air India (888-834-1407; airindia.in), Lufthansa (800-645-3880; lufthansa.com), and Delta (800-221-1212; delta.com). It can also be reached by train or road from nearby Mumbai by Sandi's shuttle bus (sandis@sandis.com).

▶ **Best Time to Visit**: March through May are Pune's hottest months. The summer, June through September, is cooled by moderate rains, resulting in pleasant daily temperatures.

▶ **Accommodations**: Homestays are the most common for students studying at RIMYI. A list is available from the Iyengar Yoga National Association of the United States (iynaus .org). Pune also has several hotels accessible through any travel agency.

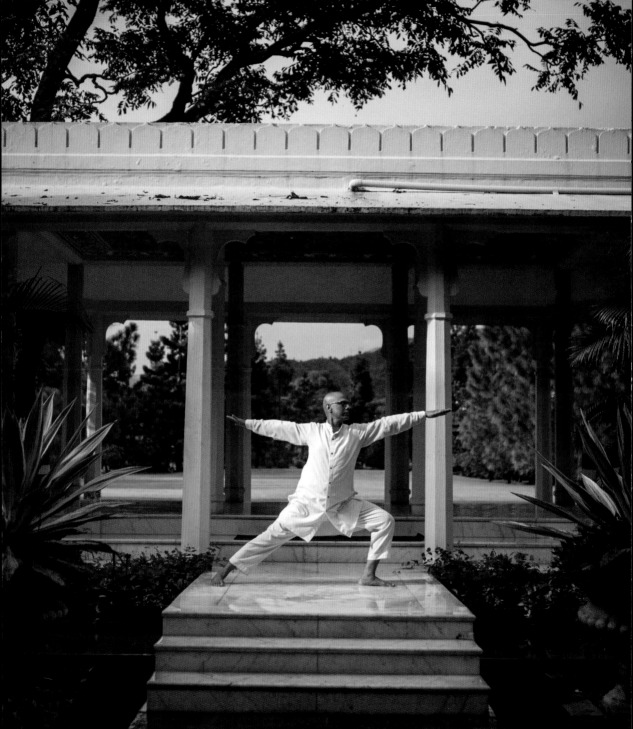

RISHIKESH

RECOMMENDED BY **Sandeep Agarwalla**

The gateway to the Himalayas. The place where the sacred Ganges breaks free from the mountains. The city that holds the title of "the birthplace of yoga" is a place of a thousand legends. One claims that the city derives its name from the story of the sage Raibhya Rishi, who was so sincere in his devotional austerities at this location that Lord Vishnu appeared to him saying, "I will reside here forever as Hrishikesh Narayan, and this place will be known as Hrishikesh." According to the Ramayana—one of the two major Sanskrit epics of ancient India—it is the city where Lord Rama performed his penance for killing King Ravana. Some people claim it is the location where Lord Vishnu defeated the powerful Veda-stealing demons Madhu and Kaitabha and returned the power of creation back to Brahma. No matter who you ask, or how far back you ask, the whole town is considered to be sacred. Even meditating here is said to lead to *moksha*, the end to the Hindu cycle of death and rebirth.

Although its rich history spans thousands of years, the West did not truly get its eyes on Rishikesh until the Beatles visited with their guru, Maharishi Mahesh, in 1968. Today the city bursts with thousands of international visitors wishing to see, learn, and grow from this sacred well. "This whole region and the river Ganga have very high spiritual powers," began Sandeep Agarwalla. "With this many ashrams, yoga, meditation centers, pilgrims, and people seeking prayers all in one place, it has a very different energy from other cities."

Despite global popularity, the city retains its yogic soul. Nonvegetarian food and alcohol are officially prohibited and the town's stone lanes and alleys have an old-world charm. Rishikesh is shaded by cool green trees and abundant nature, with the green-blue Ganges flowing strong everywhere you look. Located in the northeast of the country, it is

OPPOSITE:
The famed birthplace of yoga offers unparalleled experiences for yogis to realign with their practice, whether at renowned wellness hotels or humble dirt floor shalas.

DESTINATION 29

especially pleasant between April and August, when the rest of India is shimmering in heat. Visiting yogis will have no trouble finding a community to connect with. There are rustic, bare-floor ashrams, thick with dust and chanting voices while the clamor of horns, rickshaws, and the occasional monkey tests your discipline and focus. There are hotel-like centers, resembling small homes, demanding that their residents refrain from garlic, eggs, and worldly talk during their stay.

Then, far up in the hills, set apart from the town, almost on another plane of existence, is Ananda. Known as India's premier wellness resort, Ananda is not so much a hotel as a palace—literally, an expanse of heavenly white towers that once served as the home of the Maharaja of Garhwal. Despite this princely reputation, Ananda is a world dedicated to healing.

"When I came here, I noticed the guests were very open to the teachings I had," continued Sandeep. "They were not looking for the Western approach to yoga. They were looking for the more fundamental teachings: purity, transparency, and discipline." The spa at Ananda focuses on hatha yoga, which, according to legend, was founded by Shiva himself. For advanced practitioners, this return to classical purity can be refreshing, and for beginners it is the perfect place to learn. "We follow the Bihar school tradition," Sandeep explained. "It comes from Swami Sivananda of the Divine Life Society. Sometimes we have to remind people that this is not a sport. It's not like how you've been doing it in the West. Physical postures are easy to deal with, so people think that's the beginning and end of yoga—but it's just the tip of the iceberg. We go beyond doing asanas and complex postures. We do structured meditation and breathing exercises for the mind. This is not a retreat; that is not the idea of yoga we have. The idea is to build something you can take home with you."

Visitors to Rishikesh often come with objectives mirroring that of a pilgrimage, and this is welcomed at Ananda. "You don't just come and stay at the hotel," continued Sandeep. "You walk in with a goal, whether it's to improve your yoga, de-stress, or detox. Everyone gets an Ayurvedic analysis on arrival and, for your entire stay, all of your classes, oils used in the spa treatments, and diet are custom built around this. The goal is to take each person on a journey. Throughout the seven days, you feel a progression."

Floating in the green layer of the Himalayas, while eagles glide by and clouds wander above, Ananda offers a respite from the bustling city below, an ideal place to connect with Rishikesh's cosmic energy. "The music pavilion is a favorite of mine, with the sounds of the water flowing," reflected Sandeep. "We also have the Hava Mahal, where ceilings are high and blue and open from all sides. Everything feels airy."

Those who visit Rishikesh typically return home as different people, changed as only one can be from having connected with the source. "Those who are open and flexible have the best experiences at Ananda and in Rishikesh," Sandeep said. "You just have to allow the system to work on you. We meet people who have done yoga for many years come here and say [that it's completely different from what they've been doing at home]. It is a journey. Most of the teaching is simple guidance. We just try to put people on their personal path."

SANDEEP AGARWALLA is the head of yoga at Ananda in the Himalayas, India. After living the life of a yogi and studying at the prestigious Bihar Yoga Bharati with an MA in yoga physiology, he chose to teach in the Bihar yoga centers in different parts of India to further hone his skills. He joined Ananda in the Himalayas in 2009. With a brief sojourn internationally to set up a traditional wellness center, Sandeep returned to Ananda as the head of yoga. He has been instrumental in taking Ananda's traditional Hatha yoga and meditation practice to the next level, creating the Dhyana (self-realization) program based on traditional meditation.

If You Go

▶ **Getting There**: The nearest airport to Rishikesh is India's domestic Dehradun's Jolly Grant Airport, twenty-two miles away. Most international visitors will likely fly into Delhi or Mumbai, and then connect to Dehradun on a flight on IndiGo (+91 1246173838; goindigo.in) or SpiceJet (+91 9871803333; spicejet.com).

▶ **Best Time to Visit**: The International Yoga Festival is typically held in March. Rishikesh is very hot in late spring, but temperatures begin to drop in July with the arrival of steady monsoon rain. Autumn sees both the lowest rain and calmest temperatures.

▶ **Accommodations**: Ananda Spa is bookable at anandaspa.com. Other hotels and shalas can be found with the Uttarakhand Tourism Board at uttarakhandtourism.gov.in/destination/rishikesh.

DESTINATION

29

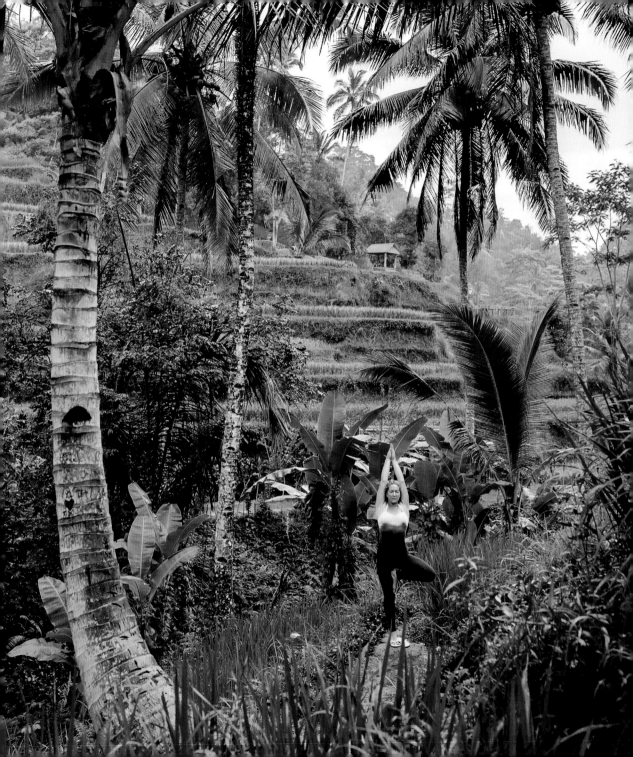

BALI

RECOMMENDED BY **Sarah Harvison**

Nestled in the Sunda Arc between the Indian and Pacific Oceans, the tiny island of Bali is one of Indonesia's crown jewels. Renowned for its rich history and artistic legacy, it is also Indonesia's only predominantly Hindu province. Its swaying palm trees, aquamarine seas, and coral sunsets have been a siren's call to soul-searchers and devoted yogis of all backgrounds since 2010, when Elizabeth Gilbert's epic *Eat Pray Love* took the Western world by storm. For Sarah Harvison, it was a trip to Bali—before the influence of *Eat Pray Love* reached a tipping point—that helped launch her love affair with yoga.

"Growing up, my mother had been a yoga teacher, but it always sort of embarrassed me," Sarah confessed. "I thought it was a little dorky. Just after graduation, I found myself living on a two-hundred-acre farm in Australia, but something wasn't right. I felt directionless, uneasy. I was searching for something, but I wasn't sure what. I had a lifelong love of movement and self-inquiry, and alone on this farm, I found myself turning again and again to the Rodney Yee yoga DVDs in the living room. Eventually, I noticed my daily practices in front of the TV were becoming less about the workout and more about something greater. I recalled that my mom, who is a mental-health nurse, used yoga for solace and stress management, and here I was at a place in my life where I needed to do some serious self-inquiry." Something clicked, and she eventually made the decision to go beyond yoga for sport and to begin yoga for spiritual practice.

"So many people go to teacher training during a really low place in their life, or when they're seeking something," reflected Sarah. "To be able to dedicate the time, you often have to be in a transitional space, and Bali has its arms wide open to you for that."

Following her realization in Australia, Sarah was eager to begin her teacher training and come away with a high degree of confidence. YogaWorks, a Los Angeles–based yoga

OPPOSITE:
With a famed tropical climate, Bali's lush jungles and warm beaches have been hosting yogis for decades.

DESTINATION

30

center that offered five-week intensive teacher trainings, had a program that fit the bill, including one with renowned teacher Ayesha Cheung. It was set to take place on a little island called Bali. "This was back when no one I knew had even heard of Bali," Sarah added. "I was essentially flying alone to the middle of nowhere."

The training was held at Pondok Pitaya on the southwestern coast of the island. The beaches are lined in glittering black sand and quiet. "I felt very welcome from the beginning," Sarah recalled. "The Balinese people and the other workshop attendees were so kind. Bali was also very easy on my recent-graduate wallet. By American standards, it was insanely affordable; you could eat incredibly delicious, fresh food for $30 a week."

At Pondok Pitaya, practice begins at 6:30 A.M. every day. "It was physically, emotionally, and spiritually demanding," Sarah continued. "But I found myself inspired by the strong, confident, and kind presence of Ayesha. One of my favorite lessons that she taught me, that I still say to myself today, is 'When head and heart are wrestling with a decision, your gut knows the answer.' So much of yoga is a metaphor for life, how to not bend too far backward or forward, but instead, be open. I discovered what my gut was trying to tell me all along: I am a whole person on my own. Bali helped me find my own voice, and yoga helped me find independence, self-inquiry, wholeness, and an element of divinity. Finding completion in who I am wouldn't have happened if I hadn't done that training."

Bali is no longer a secret. The presence of boutique hotels like W and Conrad attest to the fact that Bali has arrived as a tourist destination. International events like the Bali Spirit Festival, the Bali International Film Festival, and a plethora of year-round music, light, and religious festivals have made tourism-related business 80 percent of the Balinese economy. Its most famous event, the Bali Spirit Festival, was founded in 2008 as an international holistic health and world music event. Every spring it draws more than five thousand participants from around the world. "It's very global, like an OG Wanderlust. Often, you're practicing on a dirt floor with hundreds of other yogis, led by a teacher who doesn't speak English."

Despite the increase in traffic, Bali hasn't lost any of its famous craftsmanship and heart. Almost everyone who visits agrees that Bali boasts a special aura. "Some of my favorite things about the place are the little hidden roads and spots you can find," Sarah said. "I was walking one evening with a fellow yogi, and we found a hand-painted, little yellow sign for a restaurant. We took a turn down a cobblestone path that led us to a rice field, where we saw a little house, right in the middle of the field. There was a man playing guitar, and a woman cooking. No one else was there. They greeted us and welcomed us in, and the woman fed us an incredibly beautiful meal, while the man played alongside her. I feel like these places are hidden everywhere in Bali. Years later, I was able to find the place again—that time with my mother."

SARAH HARVISON is the manager of the global ambassador program at Lululemon and taught at the prestigious Semperviva studio in Vancouver, British Columbia, before its closure in 2020. Working with one of the most prestigious athleisure brands on the planet, Sarah seeks out community leaders and experts in the yoga community and works to integrate yoga programming and global yoga influencers into brand campaigns, cross-functional partnerships, and global events and experiences. She is also co-CEO of the #100SweatySweats Instagram challenge movement, which inspires people to stay in motion and in community for a hundred days each year.

If You Go

▶ **Getting There**: Major airlines such as Delta (800-221-1212; delta.com) and Cathay Pacific (800-233-2742; cathaypacific.com) fly directly into Bali (Denpasar). Taxis are the most common way tourists get around the island once landed.
▶ **Best Time to Visit**: Bali has a distinct dry season and wet season. April through October is best for those who want to avoid the rain.
▶ **Accommodations**: Pondok Pitaya on Balian Beach is bookable at pondokpitaya.com. The Bali Tourism Board lists a variety of other yoga-friendly hotels at thebalibible.com.

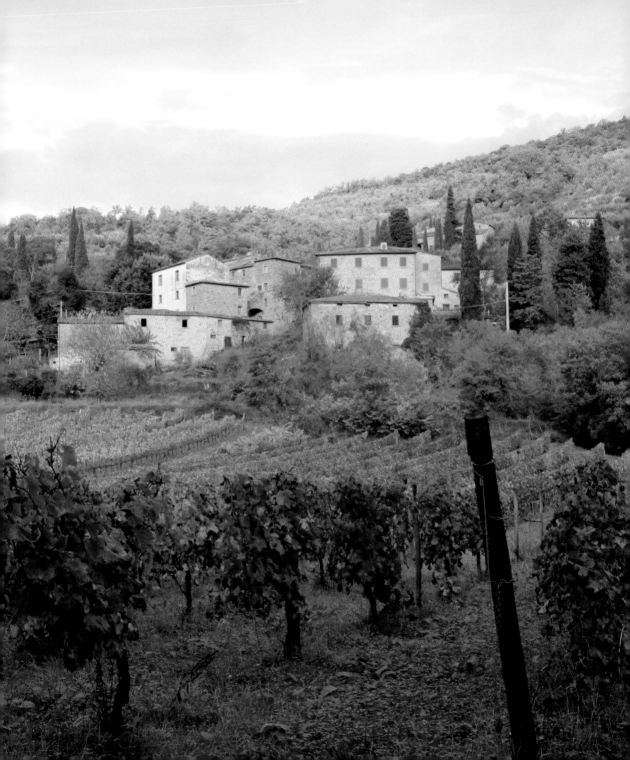

VAL DI CHIO

RECOMMENDED BY **Eli Walker**

Traditionally, alcohol and yoga do not mix. Even as yoga has spread out of Indian temples and into the West, many modern yoga retreats do not offer their guests any liquid courage.

But this is not the philosophy of a particular yoga retreat in Italy.

"I was exhausted with the male parts of yoga where they abused spiritual power and told people what to do," began Eli Walker. "The nature of most yoga classes is very militaristic. You don't ask questions, you're supposed to stay quiet, not look at anyone, blindly do what you're told, and surrender your ego until you find enlightenment. I wanted something different, something that was about connection and community.

"At its core, Drunk Yoga® is not about the asana flow. It's also not about getting wasted. It's about combining something familiar with something unfamiliar, to cultivate joy together. Most people who come to these retreats are total beginners who think they can't do any yoga at all. Then they get a glass of wine in them, and poof! Maybe they can touch their toes. When I first started, I got sizzling hate mail from a lot of purists. People said I was appropriating yoga, people thought I was debauched, just some dumb hipster from New York. There is this strict, linear vision of what yoga is—that it's for health and detoxing and mental clarity—but you get those things whenever you do any exercise. Yoga is about union and joy. I wanted to create communities, to bring people together in a place they're comfortable socializing. I wanted to turn yoga into happy hour."

There is perhaps no better place for happy hour than Tuscany. The Italian countryside is famous for its long, warm summers, gently rolling hills, and, of course, the liquid gold of its grapes. But today, it is not only a place for wine aficionados to explore the terroir that produces some of the world's most revered wines; it's also a place to connect with a radical approach to yoga at a location that has been defying conventions for centuries.

OPPOSITE:

Famiglia Buccelletti, one of Italy's oldest wineries, is one of the gems of the Tuscan countryside.

DESTINATION

31

"We host the Drunk Yoga retreat at one of the oldest wineries in Italy. Famiglia Buccelletti is also the only totally female-run winery in Tuscany," continued Eli. "Wine making is still very much a male-dominated industry. When these women first started to make wine, no one took them seriously, and their labels were changed to deny that it was made by women. This made it the perfect place to partner with for a retreat."

The Val di Chio, an area in the eastern, interior reaches of the Tuscan countryside, has been called the "Tuscan Garden of Eden." The Casali di Famiglia Buccelletti is not a hotel in the traditional sense but, instead, a meticulously preserved and restored medieval village, with many of the structures dating back to 1100 CE. Gravel roads meander past clusters of rustic brick buildings, groves of olive trees, and organic gardens bursting with tomatoes, squash, and citrus, all attended by rows of tall Italian cypresses. Wrought iron and wood doors, crystal clear fountains, and acres of grapes basking in the sun all make this little village a quintessential picture of Tuscan glory. "We're on a high hill, overlooking most of what rolls downward," Eli reflected. "A favorite thing to do is to lean back in the pool and take it all in with a glass of organic Tuscan wine in your hand. The feeling is just paradise. We do sober yoga in the morning, and then yoga with wine overlooking the hills of Tuscany in the evening. We have long, communal meals, and people have time to move slowly, explore, and connect with each other. There is also so much to see and do around here."

The Val di Chio, in addition to being one of the most agriculturally rich parts of Tuscany, is home to a brilliant walking tour. After performing asana practice with friends at the villa, visitors can stroll the green hills surrounding the winery in all directions. The trails take you past fields of sunflowers; small, friendly towns built of wood and cobble-stones (the tiny town of Cortona, where *Under the Tuscan Sun* was filmed, just so happens to be nearby); and, for fans of medieval history, the ruins of ancient castles. Archaeologists suspect that the area has been inhabited for over three thousand years; nearby Castiglion Fiorentino, which once housed Etruscans and Romans, has kept its stone-and-mortar walls almost entirely intact. The nearby underground Civic Museum of Archaeology and Excavation collects discoveries found in the Castiglion territory, and village piazza archaeologists have discovered a sacred area within the city's walls that dates back to the fifth century BCE.

"I'm a New Yorker, and New Yorkers are martyrs by nature," concluded Eli. "They just want to work hard, suffer, and not look at anybody until they die. But I didn't want to bring that to my yoga practice anymore. This is something warmer, where people can look at each other, talk to each other, talk to me, and leave happier than when they came in. Tuscany is a great place for that. I want to lift people's spirits to empower them to do the same for others. This is about warmth and community; 100 percent about sparking joy."

ELI WALKER grew up in rural Wisconsin and set flight for Manhattan when she received a scholarship to attend Tisch School of the Arts. She set out to be an actress, but it wasn't long before her passion for using performance as a tool to cultivate awareness of the physical and spiritual body led her to the art of yoga. Eli completed her five-hundred-hour RYT in Manhattan and received additional training in Iyengar, reiki, reflexology, and vipassana meditation in India during a six-month solo-backpacking trip across the country. After a severe injury in Thailand, she returned to NYC and discovered Katonah Yoga, an esoteric practice developed by Nevine Michaan, which combines hatha, sacred geometry and Taoist philosophy. Drawing from all of these experiences, Eli developed the Divine Your Story™ teaching method in 2017, and integrated theater and yoga one step further in order to make the art of joy even more accessible to the masses by creating the internationally acclaimed (albeit subversive) company Drunk Yoga and the online membership UPLIFT for virtual Drunk Yoga experiences.

If You Go

▶ **Getting There**: It's generally easiest to fly into Florence, served by Vueling (+34 931518158; vueling.com) or British Airways (800-247-9297; britishairways.com), and either book a taxi or shuttle for the two-hour drive. You can also catch a train from either Rome or Florence to the Castiglion Fiorentino station.

▶ **Best Time to Visit**: Summers are hot and mark the tourist season for Tuscany, and those who dislike rain should avoid October.

▶ **Accommodations**: The Casali in Val di Chio has numerous properties, bookable at villas.famigliabuccelletti.it.

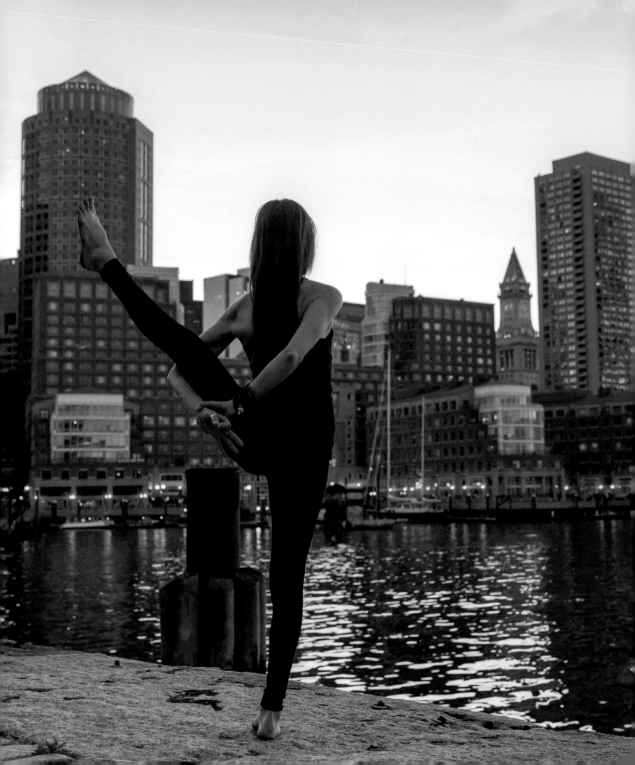

BOSTON

RECOMMENDED BY **Justine Wiltshire Cohen**

Boston, the spiritual capital of New England, is a city with symbolic significance for the development of the American consciousness. It saw the foments of the American Revolution, and holds the relics of some of the earliest forms of American culture. The city's 2.5-mile "Freedom Trail" takes you past a string of sites where America's independence was born, including the Boston Common and the Bunker Hill Monument. Although the age of colonial revolution was centuries ago, Boston remains a hub of some of the most dynamic educational, cultural, medical, and scientific activities in the United States. In sum, what happens in Boston tends to influence the rest of the country in powerful ways. This includes yoga.

Down Under School of Yoga is a collection of America's most renowned teachers who came together to form a yoga home, a place of teaching and learning. "You can find yoga almost anywhere in this country," reflected Director Justine Wiltshire Cohen. "But Boston is the intellectual yoga capital of America, boasting a cluster of illustrious lineage-based teachers as well as an equally impressive band of renegade modernists who critically examine tradition. We founded Down Under to bring them together under one roof."

The Iyengar School, offering precision and alignment, is directed by America's most senior Iyengar teacher, Patricia Walden. The Ashtanga School, with its druid-like yogis emerging out of the dawn mists to practice silently with the rising sun, is led by the burning zeal and intelligence of Sam Glannon and the mothering wisdom of orthopedic surgeon Didi von Deck, two distinguished authorized teachers in a lineage where certification can only come from India and is thus a rarity in the US. The mindful tranquility of the Restorative School owes much to the perceptive and empathic Ryan Cunningham, a veteran of the Boston yoga scene, and his "Slow Flow" mentor, the

OPPOSITE:
From the
Boston Harbor
to the Emerald
Necklace,
Boston offers
yogis a variety
of venues and
lineages to
nourish their
practice.

DESTINATION

32

147

irreverent and delightful Barbara Benagh. The school marries Natasha Rizopoulos, a national vinyasa treasure, with the dynamic and joyful yoga free-form of Jojo Reger and American champion rowing coach Marina Traub. Boston is also considered the birthplace of Power Yoga—Gregor Singleton and his wife, Claire Este McDonald, helped pioneer the aerobic style under Baron Baptiste some twenty years ago (Claire also heads up the nearby Boston Ayurveda School). This extraordinary cast of characters and sixty other teachers make up what is one of America's most esteemed faculties. "Each tradition whispers its own secrets. Each teacher works on a different aspect of the practice. The vision behind our school is allowing students access to all those traditions under one roof," reflected Justine.

From its humble beginnings in a church basement, to its position of prominence in the yoga scene today, Down Under seeks not just to hold space for most major yoga lineages, but also to create conversations between lineages, as well as coworking opportunites to solve problems in the yoga community. "We don't blend methodologies—each tradition stands in its integrity—but there is vibrant dialogue and conversation around those methodologies and the role of yoga in this current cultural context," Justine continued. "Those beautiful moments of discourse and collaboration, and sometimes respectful disagreement, are the reason the school is so exciting. For example, the issues around touch, physical adjustments, and consent inspired us hold a public forum on power dynamics with leads of all lineages discussing yoga's "dirty little secrets" and sex scandals. We created new studio protocols so students now proactively indicate their willingness to receive assists and can review a photographic manual of acceptable standard adjustments so they can understand exactly what they are consenting to."

Similarly, the studio was responsive to calls for racial justice in America by rolling out a task force to address the lack of black teachers in the yoga industry, doubling its training scholarships for black, indigenous people of color, inviting critique around making the studios more welcoming, and immediately appointing teachers of color to positions of leadership internally. When the COVID-19 virus decimated cities across America and yoga studios folded by the thousands, Down Under remained one of the only independent schools that did not fire or furlough a single teacher or manager. It rode out the crisis with directors suspending their pay rather than cutting the pay of their managers. Down Under seeks to recast what a yoga school can do—not only in its class and conversation offerings, but also in its company structure, including company governance and the treatment of its employees. "Another dirty secret of yoga is that very few teachers in America can make a sustainable income," said Justine. "Making our teachers employees, with access to sick days, health care, matching retirement, and even managerial salaries, was a big step. I have empathy for small-business owners just starting out because opening a yoga studio is hard. You try to do the right thing, but you don't always have the money. After seventeen years, we are so pleased to be able to bring these yogic concepts of sustainability off the mat and behind the scenes."

Down Under School of Yoga has three different studio locations across Boston, including Newton, Brookline, and Cambridge, and soon to be downtown. It keeps its building designs simple and clean, with walls of windows to let the world inside the room. "If you peek in, it can look very different here depending on the time of day," Justine described. "You might see Iyengar practitioners delighting in the precision and alignment of one pose at a time, using props, or rope walls or the six-foot 'horse.' Perhaps later, you'll see bodies flowing from pose to pose in lyrical, rhythmic vinyasa sun salutations. Then our power yogis look like Olympian gods, glowing with the sweat of their vigorous, raw emotional work. Or if it's slow flow, you'll witness the depth of practitioners moving so mindfully and deeply that the focus shifts to giving in and listening. In a day, you'll find the world of yoga at your feet, as if the yoga poses themselves are asking you to explore your relationship to intensity and softness.

If you head to Boston to experience Down Under, be sure to check out some of the city's other sights. History buffs will enjoy the Old South Meeting House, the largest building in colonial Boston, where citizens gathered to challenge British rule. Nature-lovers will appreciate the emerald necklace, a 1,100-acre string of grassy parks linked by sidewalks and waterways. "Crystal Lake is one of my favorites," reflected Justine. "It's in Newton and would have you thinking you're in the backcountry rather than just outside an international city. Boston is full of these quiet spaces to duck into. And then of course there are lovely beaches up in Rockport, down near Quincy, and on Cape Cod, where the Kennedys camped out. You often see beautiful outdoor beachfront yoga happening there.

"Lineage is of tremendous value in that we all stand on the shoulders of giants, but it's equally important to look at how we pass on these traditions, integrating the best of our humanity and society as we do so. This ancient tradition passed from teacher to students for ages also implies a responsibility that our choices and actions shape where yoga is headed. In the age of corporate chains and gym yoga, it can sometimes appear as if dumbed-down, dressed-up fitness classes are now confused for yoga. It's all in the marketing, right? We beg to differ. When Down Under is dubbed 'le residence' to those big models of shareholder-driven marketing, we bear that moniker with pride."

JUSTINE WILTSHIRE COHEN was born in Australia and introduced to yoga and the cultures of the East by her journalist parents, who taught English to Tibetan monks in the Dalai Lama's community. After attending law school, Justine worked in international human rights, spending "crazy hours doing good" while neglecting her own body. She decided to experiment with "cleaning house" and thus began a journey of study with many remarkable teachers of meditation, psychology, and yoga. She, like many of Down Under's other teachers, has studied with leading instructors, including Dr. Sandra Parker in Vancouver, John Schumacher in Washington, DC, and Patricia Walden in Boston. Following a stint as yoga teacher at the US Supreme Court, Justine married a Boston boy in 2003 and established Down Under in Newton Highlands the following year.

If You Go

▶ **Getting There**: Boston International Airport is served by most major carriers.
▶ **Best Time to Visit**: Boston has notoriously long, cold winters, lovely green summers, and the magical "changing colors" of autumn, which can be a wonderful time to visit.
▶ **Accommodations**: The Greater Boston Convention & Visitors Bureau (bostonusa.com) lists a number of options, from upscale luxury hotels to budget-friendly hostels.

STOCKBRIDGE

RECOMMENDED BY **Barbara Vacarr**

"I often say people coming to Kripalu are in grave danger of growing," said Barbara Vacarr, PhD. "I took a circuitous path to get here as CEO. In many ways, it's the culmination and integration of so much of what has consumed me. I grew up an ultra-orthodox Jew, but left at a young age on a path of seeking. I spent time at a Buddhist community, then a Sufi community, and came to Kripalu when it was just an ashram. It was such a strong community. But since I was leaving a strong community, it didn't call to me at that time. However, I found myself coming back; something was drawing me. Over the years, I came to understand that Kripalu is an antidote to the kind of stress and challenge that we're living in today."

The center's seeds were planted in 1960, when Amrit Desai, a disciple of revered Indian Swami Kripalu, came to Philadelphia from India. Swami Kripalu, sometimes called Bapuji ("dear father"), was a dedicated yogi whose kundalini-based teachings emphasized the cultivation of personal health, daily practice, well-being, and a virtuous character. He encouraged Amrit to share this potent form of yoga with Americans, leading him to co-found the Yoga Society of Pennsylvania and set up a residential yoga center in Sumneytown, which would come to be known as the "Kripalu Yoga Fellowship." The message resonated across the country, and the Fellowship grew. In 1983, the center found a new home in a sprawling Victorian estate in the Berkshires known as "Shadowbrook."

"What we're doing here is really about changing the world and supporting people to develop," Barbara continued. "We foster the kind of learning that makes people want to make a difference in their lives and the lives of others."

Today, to call Kripalu a "yoga center" would be a bit like calling the Pacific Ocean a pond. It is the premier East Coast destination for yogis, students of Eastern-based healing

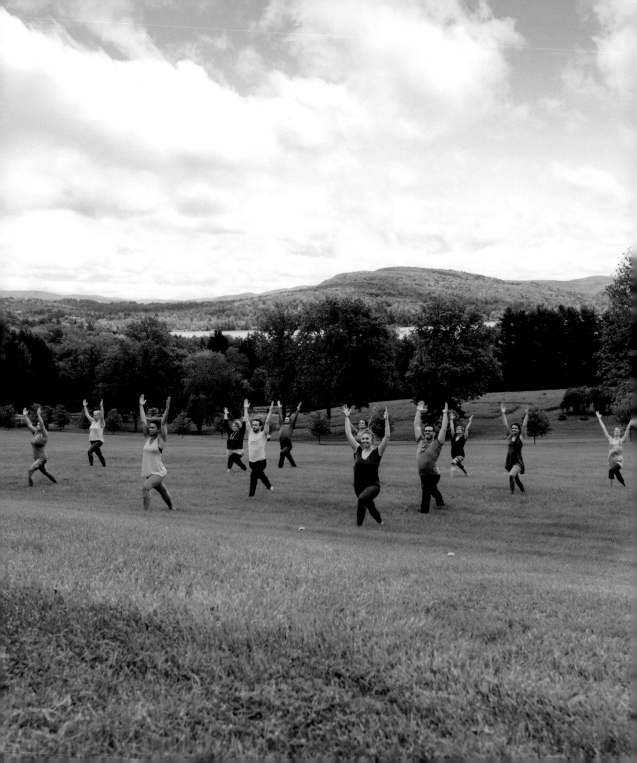

arts, and others on a path to self-discovery. It is one part hotel resort, one part health center, and one part school, hosting more than seven hundred programs a year in Ayurveda, yoga, mindfulness, and consciousness innovation. Certifications from its Schools of Yoga, Ayurveda, Integrative Yoga Therapy, and Mindful Outdoor Leadership are respected across the world. Guest presenters regularly include superstar yogis, such as Rodney Yee, Judith Hanson Lasater, and Kathryn Budig, as well as a variety of premier spiritual leaders from around the world. Whether you're just beginning yoga, are a dedicated practitioner, or are simply seeking an R&R vacation with a conscious lean, Kripalu has something for everyone.

OPPOSITE:
The Berkshires
provide a serene
setting for
practitioners
honing their skills
at Kripalu.

"We are talking about yoga with a big Y: yoga on the mat and off the mat," Barbara explained. "You don't have to be a yogi to come to Kripalu. We get all kinds of explorers here—people in life transitions, people experiencing loss, people craving nature—many of whom have never done yoga. We say, come as you are. Our ultimate goal is to foster self-compassion as a pre-req for creating more compassion in the world."

With so many programs, guests, and schools, it's hard to imagine that a typical day is possible, but the center has its own harmony. "There's a rhythm to the day," Barbara continued. "It begins with connection to self. At six A.M., we have our first practice, which, in the summer, is hosted outside with a view of our lake, the Stockbridge Bowl. We breathe, reflect, and become embodied. After this practice, we offer a silent breakfast to all guests. This takes some people by surprise, but they leave feeling like they never appreciated how important silence is. Our food gets our highest scores from guest experience. It's gluten sensitive, local, mostly vegan vegetarian, with a few meat options. So, you come in in silence to all this abundance. It changes people. You see guests sitting over their food in a different way. They are relating to their food, feeling their bodies and present to themselves. I've heard it called 'delicious contemplation.'

"Then, every day at noon, we have my favorite thing of all time: yoga dance. I cannot describe the joy and sensation of seeing this. I've watched people who tend to feel uncomfortable in their bodies get into the free flow of this; even skeptics join in. It is so joyful."

Throughout the day, programs on topics such as past-life regression, energy medicine, Ayurvedic cooking, and physical anatomy beckon the curious visitor. Another option is to leave the mansion and engage with the forests and meadows surrounding the estate. Tracking and snowshoeing are offered in the silence of winter. Autumn offers beautiful bursts of sungold and orange and red from the trees. Summer and spring are alive with

DESTINATION

33

grass and flowers. "We're surrounded by hiking trails and natural beauty," Barbara enthused. "One of my favorite places to go is the labyrinths. There's a gateway that leads to them that feels like a portal. In the first year and a half I was here, I walked them every single day. They overlook the water, and you get to feel the entire expanse of the Berkshires in this very contained space. Another wonderful place is the Swami Kripalu meditation space, located a short walk into the forest. You walk up this stepped area into what feels like a wooden enclosure. It is not fancy or polished. It's very humble and organic, like it's part of the surroundings. The other day when I was there, a beautiful red fox came to greet me. I thought it was very fortuitous."

After a day of workshops, nature, and yoga, dinner awaits guests in the main hall, followed by an evening program: often kirtan, sound bowl, or an intensely relaxing session of guided yoga nidra to help people sleep.

With such variety, it is no wonder Kripalu has become such a renowned destination for yogis across the world. Barbara summed up the center's philosophy as follows: "Everything we do is in the framework of what Kripalu knows about being human—how we use our bodies, our breath, to engage with whatever the content is. This is a place where people become activated to change the world."

BARBARA VACARR, PhD, joined Kripalu as CEO in 2016. She is a psychologist, an adult educator, and the former president and CEO of Goddard College in Vermont. Committed to learning what creates meaningful change in the world, Barbara has spent almost thirty years developing programs that support human growth and development and organizational transformation. She is a proud platinum member of the Women Presidents' Organization, founding director of the adult learning program at Lesley University, founder and senior leader of the Intergenerational Women's Mentoring Collective, and project leader for the Cambodian Youth and Missing History Project. Barbara was named one of fifty "Influencers in Aging in America" in 2015, by PBS's Next Avenue. She is a sought-after speaker and writer on topics including mindfulness, compassion, conscious leadership, and activism. Barbara and her husband of forty years are grandparents of five. She most enjoys spending time with her family.

If You Go

▶ **Getting There**: Albany, New York, is the closest airport and just over an hour's drive away. Hartford and Boston airports follow, with slightly longer drives. A shuttle can take you from the airport to Kripalu, if arranged ahead of time. A bus can also be taken from Boston or Albany to the Lenox stop in Stockbridge. For a smaller fee, a shuttle can take you to the center.

▶ **Best Time to Visit**: Stockbridge experiences the classic New England four seasons, with green springs, warm summers, colorful autumns, and powdery, chilly winters.

▶ **Accommodations**: A stay at Kripalu can be booked at kripalu.org.

DESTINATION

33

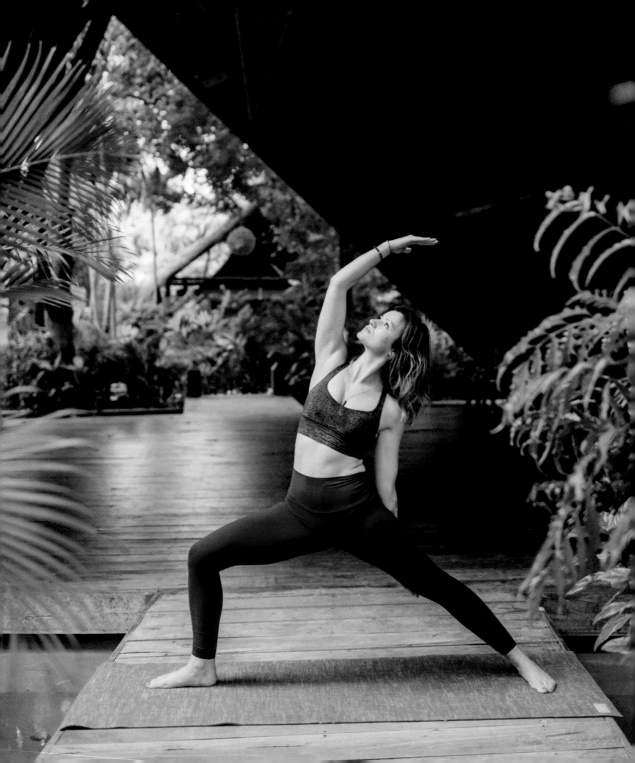

TULUM

RECOMMENDED BY **Kelli Precourt**

Kelli Precourt lives in a beachside vacation community in Florida, yet she finds special sustenance from the serenity of the beaches of Tulum, Mexico's slice of the Caribbean. "People always ask me why I travel to visit a beach when I live on a beach," Kelli began. "The energy, the people, the water, the jungle—all are very healing. Tulum is a healing place. I first visited the area as a yoga student and fell in love with the community and the culture. When I began leading retreats of my own, I thought it would be a great place to take my students. I've taken people down eight years in a row now."

Mexico's Yucatán Peninsula—the land that juts north and east into the Caribbean from Belize and Guatemala—was once the center of Mayan civilization. More recently, American and European travelers have discovered the region's rich blend of steady sunshine, unblemished beaches, and Mayan culture. One of the region's great attractions is the diving. The Mesoamerican Barrier Reef (the Atlantic's largest coral reef) lies just a few miles offshore and is home to more than five hundred fish species—both colorful reef fish and larger pelagic species (like whale sharks) are drawn to the reef. A one-of-a-kind diving experience waits inland as you leap into one of the Yucatán's many cenotes (pronounced "say-no-tays"). Cenotes are sinkholes that provide entry to extensive underground freshwater river systems; the Mayans viewed them as portals to a spiritual world below the earth. If you prefer to stay closer to the surface, snorkeling in Akumal Bay virtually guarantees an opportunity to swim alongside sea turtles.

Archaeology aficionados will want to make the two-hour trip inland to the spectacular ruins at Chichen Itza, one of the centers of Mayan domain a thousand years ago. The ruins at Tulum, overlooking the Caribbean, offer an excellent (and much closer by) primer to Mayan culture. The site is surrounded by a thick rock wall (*Tulum* means "wall" in Mayan)

OPPOSITE:
In Tulum,
the lush jungles
of the Sian
Ka'an Biosphere
Reserve meet
powdery
Caribbean
beaches,
providing
an idyllic
backdrop
for a wellness
retreat.

DESTINATION

34

and rests on a bluff thirty feet above the sea. Carvings of plumed serpents (representative of the god Kukulkan and a common Mayan design motif) grace several structures. Large flesh-and-blood iguanas laze about the rock walls.

Tulum is the gateway to the 1.3 million-acre Sian Ka'an Biosphere Reserve, which extends along the coast to the Belizean border. It's home to more than 340 bird species, endangered jaguars, and deserted, palm-tree-fringed beaches that have changed little since the Spanish conquest. Small, eco-conscious lodges dot the rough road that cuts through the reserve. This is where you'll find Maya Tulum Resort and Spa, the site of Kelli's retreat. Guests can opt for either beachside or garden-facing cabanas. Meals are taken in the resort's seaside restaurant. "The food is fantastic, all made from scratch, with nothing processed," Kelli continued. "There are lots of fresh fruits, smoothies, and even breakfast nachos. It's vegetarian-oriented, though fish is an option several nights."

Kelli's Tulum retreats are open to all levels of practitioners, and participation in sessions is optional—after all, this is also a Mexican beach vacation! The morning session begins shortly after sunrise. "Participants can join us for thirty minutes of silent meditation before I lead them through a vigorous vinyasa flow session," Kelli described. "Since I teach traditional yoga, I bring in some chanting. Then we break for breakfast. It's usually very leisurely, a chance for people to get to know each other better. Then there's a block of free time. Some will go to visit the ruins. Others might do more exercise, or sign up for a massage or other treatment. [Maya Tulum offers a range of bodyworks, including Mayan specialties like the cocoa balm wrap; yoga sessions are also available for guests not participating in a retreat.] And, of course, there's the beautiful beach and warm, crystal-clear Caribbean to enjoy. It's great to see people sipping coconut water from real coconuts! There's a late-afternoon restorative practice that's movement oriented but breath driven. Then we head from the yoga studio to the dining hall."

A wellness ritual with a distinctly Mexican flavor is the Temazcal, a sweat bath ceremony. Anthropologists believe that it was developed in Mesoamerica as a therapeutic practice to treat the sick and aid women in childbirth. Today, the ritual is also performed to provide cleansing and restorative balancing of mind, body, and spirit. Maya Tulum has a dedicated Temazcal, where participants are guided through a series of four meditations. "It's a bit scary at first," Kelli explained. "You enter this closed space and sit in a circle in the dark. There's a shaman present to guide you. It's like a rebirthing. You talk through your fears and resentments, the elements in your life that are keeping you from being the best you can be." A seaside meditation labyrinth is available for those preferring open-air contemplation.

A chance to partake of the Temazcal and practice yoga in a milieu of rich Mayan culture is one of the appeals of a Tulum retreat. For Kelli, the attraction is simpler. "The stillness and quietness of sunrise on that beach stays with me," she reminisced. "It's a reminder that life is precious and that we need to slow down and be aware of what's around us."

KELLI PRECOURT has over twenty years' experience working in the health and fitness industry as a personal trainer, certified spinning instructor, US Olympic athlete (1996; field hockey), and yoga instructor. After vacationing along the Florida Panhandle for years, Kelli felt as though something was missing . . . a yoga scene! So, in 2006, she opened Balance Health Studio with the intention of offering yoga and also providing a place where health and fitness could become a lifestyle. She also created one of the Panhandle's few yoga teacher training programs. Yoga is more than just a physical practice for Kelli; she translates yoga philosophy into a lifestyle, with a special emphasis on daily gratitude.

If You Go

▶ **Getting There**: Tulum is roughly a 1.5 hours' drive from Cancun, which is served by many major carriers. Shuttles are available.

▶ **Best Time to Visit**: Retreats are held throughout the year at Maya Tulum. Summers are uncomfortably warm for most tastes, and there's always the chance of hurricanes in the early fall. March and April are the driest months. Kelli holds her retreats in November (see her schedule of retreats at balance30a.com).

▶ **Accommodations**: Maya Tulum Retreat and Spa (888-515-4580; mayatulum.com) offers a range of comfortable accommodations and excellent food on the shores of the Caribbean. As mentioned above, there are a number of other eco-lodges offering yoga retreats in the region.

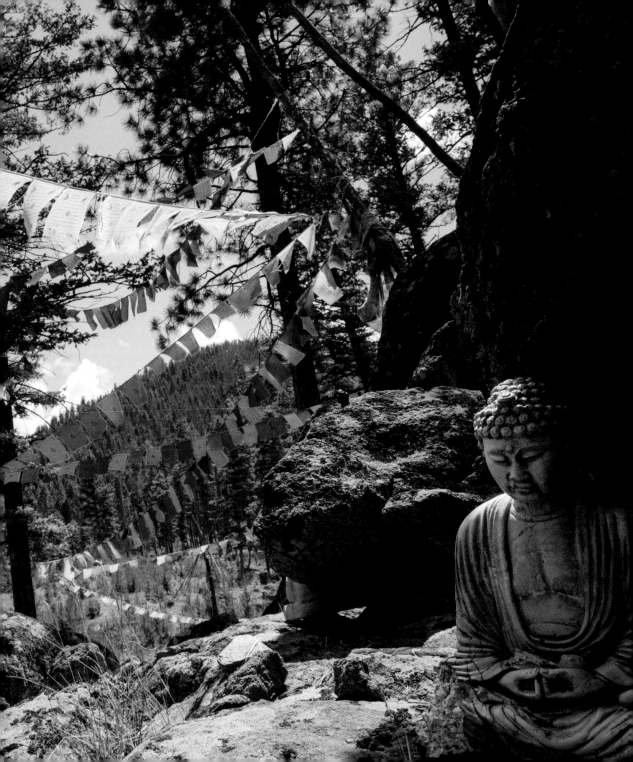

HELENA

RECOMMENDED BY **Nat Kendall**

When asked how he found yoga, Nat Kendall likes to say that he was born into it without knowing. "I was born and raised in Montana, where you're immersed in nature—the vastness of the beautiful landscape. I grew up hunting and fishing, connecting to nature and life in a very intimate way. This connection to nature, relating to the larger world, is the very definition of yoga. In this way, the state of Montana is the state of yoga.

"Most of my teaching has been in San Francisco, but five years ago I decided to make a little pilgrimage back to Montana. There was something in me that wanted to share the beauty of this state through the lens of yoga. I'd heard good things about Feathered Pipe Ranch and stopped by to visit. I sat down with India Supera, the owner, at a cabin by the lake. I didn't know it at the time, but the conversation was part of India's interview process. At the end she said, 'I think you're a good fit for this place. We'd like to invite you.' The next year, I put out an invitation to a Montana retreat to my students. I had so many people say, 'I've always wanted to explore Montana, now I can do it in the context of a yoga retreat.' Whenever I draw in that first breath of mountain air, I get a feeling unlike anywhere else. Now I get to share that feeling."

Feathered Pipe Ranch rests near Montana's capital city of Helena, in the heart of the Northern Rockies, not far from the Continental Divide. The clearing in the millions of acres of forested mountains has hosted yoga and conscious living retreats since 1975. Feathered Pipe, as it exists today, stems largely from the vision of India Supera, who landed in Montana in the early 1970s after walking around India for a year and a half in search of a guru and finally studying with Satya Sai Baba. Supera stayed in Montana longer than she had planned to help nurse a friend, Jermain Duncan, who'd been diagnosed with cancer. When Duncan passed away, she willed Supera the Feathered Pipe

OPPOSITE:
For Nat Kendall,
the state of
Montana is
the state of
yoga . . . and is
best experienced
at Feathered
Pipe Ranch.

DESTINATION

35

161

Ranch. Supera offered the ranch to Sai Baba, but he encouraged her to create an educational center. The early years were difficult, but she persevered. Over forty-plus years, she offered thousands of health, wellness, and yoga retreat attendees "the beauty and serenity of Nature and food for the mind, body and soul." (Sadly, India passed away in 2019.)

The special qualities of a trip to Feathered Pipe Ranch become evident before one even reaches the property. "You fly into Helena, and within twenty minutes, you're in the middle of nowhere, journeying into the mountains," Nat continued. "You're on a paved road for ten miles, then a dirt road, then you're winding up a rutted-out path in a little narrow drainage. You turn a corner and there's this oasis. There are sprawling lawns overlooking a lake, with glass-domed yurts, teepees, and other accommodations overlooking the scene. There's also a beautiful main lodge that was once a hunting lodge, which gives you a taste of the quintessential Montana experience. The ranch tucks up against a national forest, cottonwoods, pines, and quaking aspens, so it's all very wild."

A number of different yoga practices are explored at Feathered Pipe, including Bhakti, the focus of the retreat that Nat leads. "Bhakti yoga is about a connection to something bigger than our small minds can sometimes fathom. It's a path home to remembering how interconnected we are with the magnificence all around us," he explained. "I'm a lifelong musician, so we incorporate mantras, storytelling, and chanting in addition to the more physical yoga practices to really reawaken the heart. Bhakti is incredibly powerful; I've seen so many people find their joy again and uplift their spirits through this practice. We chant our hearts out on my retreats!"

The daily offerings at Feathered Pipe are relaxed enough to allow participants to enjoy the special Big Sky amenities. "We usually start around 7:30 with a two-hour session of meditation and asana flow," Nat described. "Then there's a break for brunch, followed by free time to hike, read by the lake, or take a canoe out for a paddle. Lunch is available mid-day, and then you have a few more hours to frolic in the woods. There's another practice session at 4:30, followed by dinner. After dinner you have the option to hang by the campfire, enjoy some s'mores, and sing mantras as the stars come out. One day during the retreat, I take the whole group for a rafting trip on the Missouri River. An amazing nonprofit environmental group guides us down the mellow rapids on a collection of rafts, kayaks, and SUPs [standup paddleboards]. There's a chance to do some agate hunting and cliff jumping, and we have a picnic dinner in a cottonwood grove at sunset. The

Missouri is a famous trout stream, and we'll see fly anglers in action, another classic Montana activity."

As one would expect at such a special place, retreats with Nat at Feathered Pipe end with a distinctive twist. "There's a rock outcropping just above the ranch known as the *stupa*," Nat described. "There's a sprawling collection of Buddhas and prayer flags that have been there for decades, and the outcropping is high enough for the mountain breezes to blow through. At the end of our stay, we walk up as a group to add flags with our prayers to the collection. There are lots of tears, cheers, and laughter. I remind everyone that their prayer will always be blowing in the mountain breezes and will find them in times of need or when they forget their connection to this world."

NAT KENDALL is a San Francisco–based yoga teacher, world music recording artist, surfer, and devoted student of yoga. A Montana native, Nat shares his wisdom of the teachings in a heartfelt and grounded way that will easily awaken beginners and re-inspire longtime practitioners. Instantly accessible and relevant to our modern times, the grace of Nat's teachings pours through in tangible practices, tools, techniques, and insights that are sure to enlighten your spiritual path and yogic journey. His devotion-filled classes are invigorating and simultaneously nurturing as he creates a space for anyone to safely explore the deep benefits of the practice.

If You Go

▶ **Getting There**: Feathered Pipe Ranch is just outside Helena, Montana, which is served by several carriers, including Delta (800-221-1212; delta.com), United (800-241-6522; united.com), and Alaska (800-252-7522; alaskaair.com).

▶ **Best Time to Visit**: Retreats are held at Feathered Pipe Ranch from June through September. Visit featheredpipe.com for a schedule of classes.

▶ **Accommodations**: There are a variety of lodging options at Feathered Pipe Ranch, including rooms in the main lodge as well as several cabins, yurts, teepees, deluxe wall tents, and regular tents. Packages include all meals and use of ranch amenities.

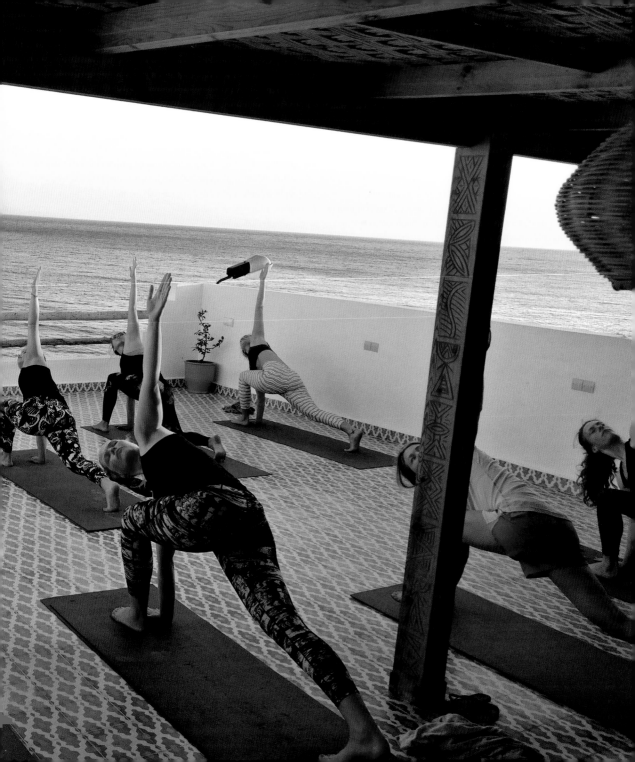

TAGHAZOUT

RECOMMENDED BY **Fenny Ramp**

Resting at the fulcrum between Europe and northern Africa, colorful Morocco has long enticed adventurous travelers. Roughly the size of California, Morocco is a land of tremendous contrasts, a place where snowcapped mountains rise from the edges of an inhospitable desert, where millennium-old neighborhoods survive in the midst of modern cityscapes. Morocco boasts over 1,200 miles of coastline. That, combined with its reputation for permissiveness toward *alternative* lifestyles (furthered by extended visits by writers like William S. Burroughs and Paul Bowles and musicians like the Rolling Stones), has made the Moroccan coast a magnet for hippies and itinerant surfers. Many were drawn to Taghazout.

"We know that surfers started visiting Taghazout in the sixties and, if you speak with the locals, it was a pretty frontier hippie front," Fenny Ramp began. "There were lots of camper vans and tents as people just chilled out on the beach for months at a time. Although the crossover between yoga and surfing hadn't really happened back then, it's likely that some of the travelers who came through would have been practicing some form of meditation and exercise routines, even back then."

Fenny came to Taghazout to get a break from the rigors of academia. "As an architectural historian, I was working at an architectural office and doing research for a professor at the University of Amsterdam. It was all very exciting, but there was also a lot of pressure and stress. I needed a break. Yoga was always a practice that helped me cope with my stress. I did my teacher training because it was always my dream to pass on what I learned from this beautiful practice. I decided to quit both my jobs and look for a place where I could teach yoga for at least a year, preferably a place where there was a nice climate and other activities to do. That's when I thought about Morocco. I'd been on a surf

OPPOSITE:
In Taghazout,
yogis and
surfers coexist
peacefully with
Berber culture.

DESTINATION

36

and yoga holiday a year before and I was very surprised by how much I liked the vibes in the Taghazout/Tamraght area. I always knew I would come back, but I never expected to come back and live here and maybe never leave. It's truly a magical place."

Yoga—and for that matter, surfing—may seem somewhat inconsistent with the mores of an Islamic country; after all, there's so much tight clothing and exposed skin. The residents of Taghazout, however, are generally not judgmental. "The Moroccan people are extremely friendly and welcoming, and that's certainly one of the appeals of the place," James Bailey, the co-owner of Surf Berbere said. "They can be tough negotiators on a business deal, but if you speak to someone for five minutes on the beach or in a café, they'll invite you to dinner in their home. I also like the fact that a town like Taghazout is still taking shape—it's not quite the finished article. There's a charm to that. I love the amazing smells, the year-round sunny, warm weather, how people are dressed differently, and the great waves.

"In Western countries we are so used to yoga at the moment," Fenny continued. "It's getting more popular every year. For Moroccan people, this is not at all the case. Even though they are getting more familiar with yoga (many surf camps are offering yoga as a beneficial addition to surfing), it hasn't yet grown in popularity with the locals. Nevertheless, they are never judgmental about it. They seem to enjoy seeing the tourists going into 'strange poses' and walking around with the funny mats."

Surfing and yoga go hand in hand around Taghazout, and practice sessions tend to run on either side of optimal surf conditions. "During peak season we run a morning class from 7:30 A.M. until 8:30 A.M., giving guests enough time to grab some food and a towel before heading out surfing," Fenny described. "We then have our sunset yoga class from 6:30 P.M. until 7:30 P.M., which combines dynamic yang and soothing yin poses. It's the perfect combination to open up the body and tackle the muscle strain that comes with surfing every day, while soothing the nerves to prepare the guests for a good night of sleep. The classes are suitable for all levels; moving in a slow pace makes it possible to go through the essentials of each yoga pose so that guests can practice them in a safe way. The sunset yoga is always a pleasure. Our open-air shala has an amazing view over the ocean where the sun sets. Not only is the view great, but it's also the best time of the day to do yoga since the sun is not that strong. Guests often stay after class to have a chat and enjoy the view together while sipping a traditional Moroccan mint tea. This is also a great moment for the yoga teacher to get to know the guests on a personal level."

Experienced surfers visiting Taghazout will find a seemingly endless selection of right-hand breaking waves to challenge their skills. Surf Berbere has accomplished teachers on hand to help beginners successfully ride waves.

A day at Surf Berbere ends with dinner on the resort's rooftop terrace. "The most famous dish in Morocco is the tajine, and it's incredibly versatile," Fenny said. "It's essentially an upside-down, dome-shaped casserole. The beauty of the casserole is that it retains the moisture but seems to spread the flavors from the core outward. A particular favorite uses dates, onions, and raisins in the core, surrounded by a mound of potatoes, cauliflower, courgettes [zucchini], and carrots in a stack. Moroccans are also famous for their salads. One of the most simple and delicious salads is their carrot and orange salad. It really only works by having fantastically fresh produce."

FENNY RAMP is a classically trained ashtangi yogi who completed her training in her native Amsterdam. She is a head yogi at Surf Berbere. Fenny believes that mind and body are interconnected, and strives to get to know her students to help them reach their goals.

If You Go

▶ **Getting There**: Most guests fly into Agadir, which is roughly an hour's drive south of Taghazout. Agadir is served by many carriers from Europe, including Ryanair (ryanair.com) and EasyJet (easyjet.com).
▶ **Best Time to Visit**: Taghazout is blessed with consistent weather and surf throughout the year. It's a bit cooler in the winter, and a bit more humid in the summer.
▶ **Accommodations**: There are a number of options designed for yogis and surfers in Taghazout, including Surf Berbere (+212 528200290; surfberbere.com).

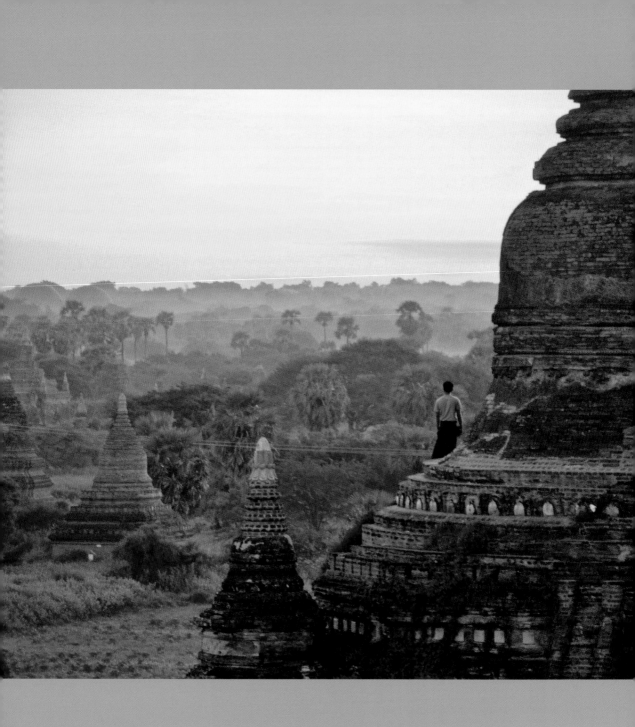

BAGAN

RECOMMENDED BY **Josh Summers**

In Myanmar, mindfulness meets action. The country's development of vipassana meditation and preservation of the Buddhist way of life runs deep. In the late nineteenth century, thousands of Buddhist monks, especially Ledi Sayadaw, empowered Burmese laypeople with education and meditation practices to fight British colonial rule, protect the *sasana* (the teachings of the Buddha), and thwart Christian takeover of the country. This sparked the global vipassana movement, which blazed across the globe through the work of mid-twentieth-century monks U Ba Khin and Mahāsi Sayādaw, who developed the meditation practices that would come to define the "mindfulness movement" in the West. "There's a continuity between traditional Indian yogic practices and Buddhist ones in Burma," posited Josh Summers. "When a meditator goes on retreat, they are actually called a yogi. One really appreciates how the physical asanas are simply a preparation for working with the mind and the developing realization of inner freedom."

The former British colony is a proud hub of Buddhism, though not always as peaceful as its monks are often characterized. The country has seen extreme human rights violations, especially against its Rohingya Muslim minority population. Despite this political strife, the protected 26-square-mile UNESCO World Heritage Site of Bagan along the Irrawaddy River remains a hub of profound Buddhist history, and a meaningful place to connect to the spiritual and philosophical practices of yoga's Buddhist roots. "It's a broad plateau, really," Josh continued, "a plain, that is studded with about three to four thousand temples and pagodas. To borrow a phrase from the anthropologist Amitav Ghosh, you feel like you're stepping into an 'antique land.' When I first got here, one of my teachers (Steven Armstrong) told me, 'When you see the monks and nuns walking off in the morning down by the river, begging for their meals, in a way you are seeing people

OPPOSITE:
The colorful,
temple-lined
horizon of
Bagan offers
viewers a chance
to see the history
of Buddhism
and Hinduism
in a new way.

DESTINATION

37

who have been walking this path since the Wheel of Dharma first spun into motion. There is an unbroken chain of tradition connecting all generations of practitioners to the very source of the Buddha himself.' It gives you shivers."

In the Bagan Archaeological Zone, for a reasonable fee, tourists have the freedom to explore the area at their leisure. One notable perk is that, unlike most major sacred sites on the globe, tourists only occasionally suffer the hard sell of cheap postcards and trinkets. Most of your neighbors will be warm and friendly laypeople, or peaceful monks. "I got up early each morning and took a donkey-driven cart to the various temples I wanted to see," Josh recalled. "The temples are dedicated to various royal family members or gods. Some of them were built before the eleventh century, when the king converted to Buddhism. Some are Hindu. Others are a blend of both religions; and many temples display artifacts of indigenous beliefs prior to the arrival of Hinduism and Buddhism. Entering each temple—dusty, musty, and modestly preserved—was like entering a portal and I would be mesmerized by their ineffable serenity and solemnity. I felt plugged into a primary artery of Buddhism's lifeblood."

The temples of Bagan take on a new dimension when viewed from above, and hot air balloon riding is a popular pastime here. "At the time, I was pretty tight on funds," Josh described. "And back then, in 2005, it was $250 for a half hour. I had just come from a two-month silent meditation retreat, so that was a pretty massive stretch for me. But I had a friend who said I simply had to do it; he even offered to loan me the money. The balloon rides happen at sunset or sunrise, and I opted for the sunrise. It started with croissants and coffee, which felt like such a luxury. Then you essentially rise into the sky with the sun and float among the temple tops. It just magnifies the panoramic awesomeness of that area. At ground level you can see there's a lot around, but then you get up, and see this grandeur. It's unlike anything I've seen anywhere else in the world."

Ashrams, shalas, and monasteries abound for a variety of Hindu, Buddhist, or nonde-nominational yogic travelers, and it's easy to pick and choose your own program. "You can go completely by yourself," Josh said. "I traveled to Bagan, carrying with me a painful, personal loss. But watching the sun come up and down from these hundreds of years-old temples, and realizing that my unique suffering was just a drop in this giant ocean of suffering that all humans experience, and knowing there is this container of teachings called the Dharma that will lift us out of the pain if we are willing to listen . . . all of that comes together in Bagan. I was so moved by the spirit and generosity of the teaching I got there.

The Burmese have such a strong sense of devotion in their practice. It's an honor to see how they preserve the path and to be able to walk with them for a few steps of the journey."

JOSH SUMMERS is an E-RYT500 yoga teacher, Lic. Ac., and founder of Summers School of Yin Yoga. He studied yin yoga with Paul Grilley and Sarah Powers, and Iyengar yoga with James Murphy. He also spent several years traveling in India, Taiwan, and Burma where he studied both yoga and meditation, primarily in the Theravada Buddhist lineages with Rodney Smith, the late Sayadaw U Pandita, and Ajahn Amaro. With *Yoga Journal*, he produced an online course called "Yin Yoga 101: The Benefits of Slowing Down" and conducted featured dialogues on meditation and spirituality for MeaningofLife.tv. He has been published in *Mindfulness and Performance* (2016, Cambridge University Press), a collection about how performers, coaches, and athletes can use mindfulness to achieve peak performance and improve personal well-being, based on the "Mindfulness and Performance" course that he co-designed and co-taught in the School of Education at Boston University. He co-authored *The Buddha's Playbook: Strategies for Enlightened Living* (2011) with Michael Brooks and *The Power of Mindfulness: Mindfulness Meditation Training in Sport* (Springer International Publishing, 2018), with Amy Baltzell.

If You Go

▶ **Getting There**: Most international travelers will have an easier time flying to Yangon Airport in Central Myanmar, served by Emirates (800-777-3999; emirates.com) and Cathay Pacific (800-233-2742; cathaypacific.com). From there, a bus ride to Bagan is about ten hours. If you arrive in Mandalay Airport in North Myanmar, served by Myanmar National Airlines (+95 1378603; flymna.com), the bus ride takes half the time, but your flight itinerary will likely be more complicated unless you are coming from Asia.

▶ **Best Time to Visit**: Bagan is fairly hot all year, with the hottest months being March and April. The cooler months from October to February are preferable.

▶ **Accommodations**: Many hotels cater to tourists in Bagan. A good list can be found with the Ministry of Health and Tourism at tourism.gov.mm/bagan.

DESTINATION

37

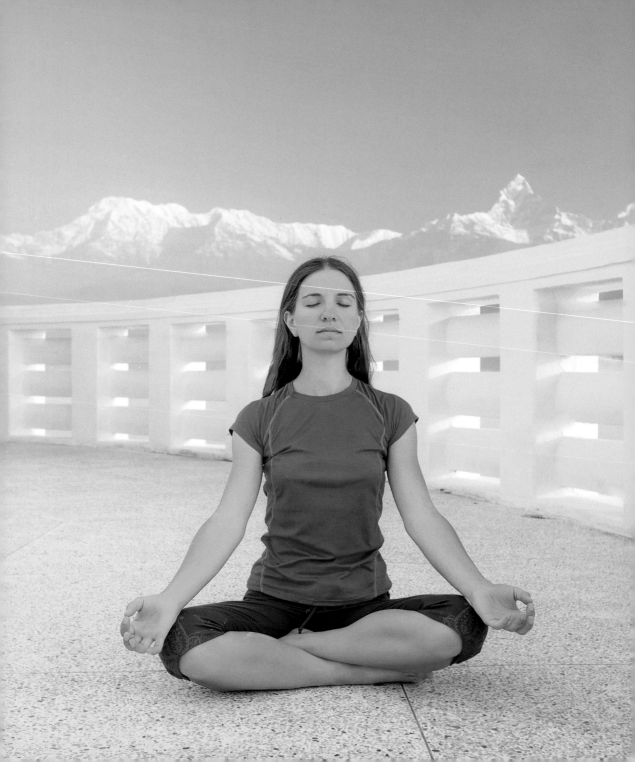

POKHARA

RECOMMENDED BY **Joaquin Gomez Picca**

At the crossroads of Buddhist and Hindu culture, Nepal has played host to seekers of both spiritual and geographic heights for centuries. Ever since Western hippies trekked into the country in the late 1960s—allured by the cheap lodging, welcoming spirituality, and wild-growing (but now illegal) marijuana—it has been a global contender for the title of "the real Shangri-La." The home of the tallest mountain in the world also boasts the birth site of Siddhartha (better known as "Buddha"), and you may even hear the occasional claim that Nepal is yoga's original home.

Yoga centers are abundant in Thamel, the tourist district in the capital city of Kathmandu. Visitors preferring a more relaxing venue can check out Dwarika's Resort, a pillar of medicinal luxury thirty miles from the Tibetan border, complete with color therapy chambers and a Himalayan rock salt *house*. A visitor with a large lung capacity can even opt for a yoga trek through the base camps of Everest.

For more back-to-basic retreats, however, yogis are encouraged to head toward the interior. "I arrived in Kathmandu and took a bus to Pokhara," said Joa Gomez Picca. "It's in the middle of the country, so we were driving through the middle of the mountains for eight hours. I remember thinking, *If this bus moves two meters to the left, we're dead.* When I arrived in Pokhara, I remember seeing cows hanging out in the street. I'm from Argentina, so it reminded me a little of the country there. I felt really grounded immediately. Pokhara is busy, but it doesn't feel big." At Rishikul Yogashala in Pokhara, a descendant of the eponymous studio from Rishikesh, Joa began training. "After I arrived, first thing in the morning, I opened the window of my room, and there was the same picture of the Himalayas—the photo that brought me there, the photo I assumed was photoshopped—right in front of me. There was so much energy. I had this overwhelming sense that I was in the right place. From that moment, I fell

OPPOSITE:
In Nepal, the
birthplace of
Siddhartha,
yogis can
meditate on
the terraces
of the Pokhara
Shanti Stupa
overlooking
the powerful
Himalayas.

DESTINATION

38

in love with the country." At Rishikul, Joa's training involved a five A.M. wake-up call, a 5:30 A.M. ashtanga asana, followed by lessons in pranayama, hatha yoga, meditation posture clinics, anatomy, and various workshops on chair yoga, power yoga, Ayurveda, Indian history, and philosophy. "It was a total of six to seven classes every day. I'm a person who needs to have a schedule, so I loved this. It makes you feel organized. It helps push you further.

"On one of our days off, the school visited the Shanti Stupa, Pokhara's biggest Buddhist temple. You get in a boat and ride across the lake for about ten to fifteen minutes. Then you arrive on the other side and walk about half an hour up a small hill. You can see all of Pokhara from above. The temple is beautiful, lots of prayer flags, of course, and the monks are very kind."

Those looking to explore Nepal's historical relationship with Buddhist Tibetan refugees can visit nearby Tashi Ling. "It's very eye-opening," Joa continued. "The town is not massive—you wouldn't go there and [be amazed by] the buildings. But the people talk to you, especially the older people. They can tell you so many things about the transition from China. It was so enlightening to have direct contact with them, rather than just reading something on Google or watching something about Tibetan refugees on TV."

Any trip to Nepal would be incomplete without a trek into the snowcapped mountains; the only question is how far you are willing to go. "During my training, we visited Sarangkot, which is right next to Pokhara," Joa recalled. "You can hike there around the mountains and even paraglide if you're not afraid of extreme heights. We slept at the foot of the mountain and, in the morning, climbed up and did yoga with the sunrise." Australian Base Camp is also nearby, a village that marks the starting point of the famous Annapurna trek, where, on a clear day, you have a famous view of the Himalayan Mountains. "It's run by this Tibetan family," Joa added. "They welcomed us inside, and I sat on the floor with the grandmother and helped her grind spices to make chai.

"Nepal has this way of bringing you back to being human. In Western countries, we've become so used to technology, living busy lives, planning and scheduling things a month out. Here, there's no plan. Of course, as a tourist, you go with a plan, but your schedule is not as strict once you show up. You can get a little frustrated. Maybe things aren't open when you want them to be because the owner got asked by his neighbor to take the cows home, so he's not there. At the same time though, this way of living is more human, more natural. The human-to-human connection flourishes, as opposed to when we are in our busy little bubbles.

"One more thing," Joa added. "I want to say that the people in Nepal are among some of the happiest people in the world. They are full of joy. Maybe it's from the culture, I honestly don't know. But they aren't pushy. They are never trying to sell you something. It is heaven to be around that."

JOAQUIN GOMEZ PICCA, better known on Instagram as @joayoga, has always been connected with movement. An ex-athlete and musician, he enjoys combining physical exercise with inner self-discovery. Joa has studied traditional as well as contemporary yoga in Nepal and India, and focuses deeply on alignment, the key for developing a safe and lasting practice. Growing up in Ibiza, Joa always had a deep connection with nature and spirituality. His love for the practice has brought him to share his knowledge with others, and he believes sharing is the most valuable and beautiful aspect of humanity. He is a certified Yoga Alliance Continuing Education Provider and an E-RYT 200 certified teacher. Joa covers a variety of styles—ashtanga vinyasa, power flow, vinyasa, hatha yoga, and restorative—in his online classes at joayoga.com, retreats in Croatia, and teacher trainings in Nepal.

If You Go

▶ **Getting There:** Fly into Tribhuvan International Airport in Kathmandu, served frequently by Nepal Airlines (nepalairlines.com.np; +977 14220757). From there, you can make a connecting flight to Pokhara's small regional airport on Yeti Airlines (+977 14465888; yetiairlines.com) or Buddha Air (+977 15521015; buddhaair.com), but most people catch a tourist bus in Kathmandu's Thamel district (no advanced reservation necessary) and enjoy the eight-hour mountain drive to Pokhara.

▶ **Best Time to Visit**: September through November is considered peak tourist season and also has the best weather. Summers are humid, hot, and quite rainy, especially July.

▶ **Accommodations**: Rishikul Yogashala (+91 9018860899; rishikulyogshala.com) welcomes yoga students on teacher training programs. Luxury hotels or simple village homestays are bookable through the Nepal Tourism Board at welcomenepal.com.

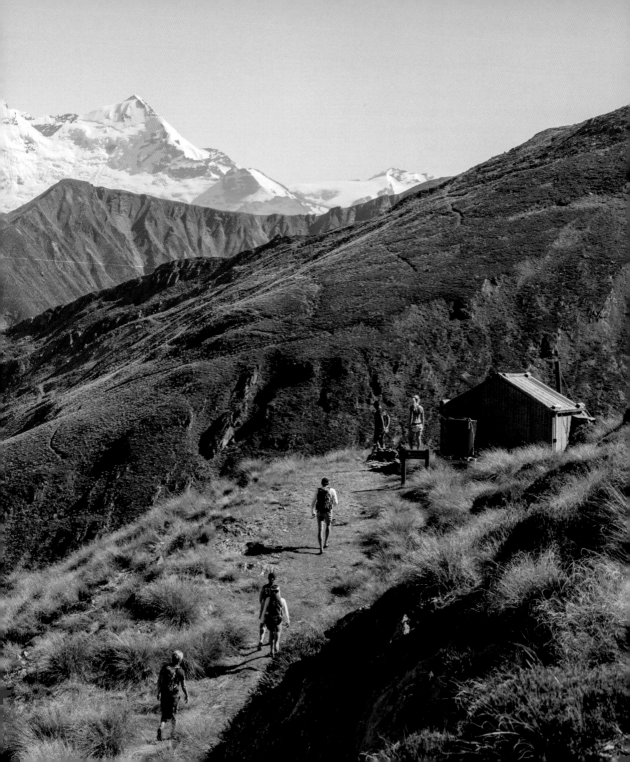

GLENORCHY

RECOMMENDED BY **Damian Chaparro**

Aro Ha Wellness Retreat, which opened its doors on the shores of Lake Wakatipu on New Zealand's South Island in 2014, was conceived some seven thousand miles away and over a decade ago. "I'd been leading yoga retreats in California," Damian Chaparro began. "I noticed that taking yourself out of your normal world, dedicating an allotment of time to a teacher or process, seemed to always increase the amplitude of students' experience, as opposed to taking a little time on the weekend. After working at the ashram, I created a wellness pop-up called Chrysalis Retreats. We wanted to offer our guests a variety of exceptional locations to visit. Traveling globally and looking for locations to host events, I noticed that very few retreat centers were addressing wellness from a holistic angle top to bottom—from program structure to food to how waste was dealt with. I began wondering what the next generation of retreat centers might look like, how they could become more sustainable, localized, and in touch with the environment.

"I shared my vision with some friends, Chris and Beth Madison. They were intrigued, and in October of 2010, we partnered to create what is now called Aro Ha. New Zealand was on the list of possible locations from the beginning. I'd never been, but once I visited, I loved the people and culture. I spent six months, mostly on the North Island, scouting locations; we thought we'd land there. But when I got to the South Island, I was blown away. I'm still enamored with the snowcapped mountains, glacially formed valleys, and long views over open spaces. Eventually we landed on a piece of land on Lake Wakatipu."

Peter Jackson's Lord of the Rings trilogy showed the world what most Kiwis already knew: The southwestern region of New Zealand's South Island is an area of incomparable natural beauty. (Moviegoers may recognize many backdrops from Middle-earth upon touching down in Glenorchy. Indeed, many scenes were filmed

OPPOSITE: At Aro Ha, guests are treated to a thoughtfully structured holistic wellness experience, including a carefully researched menu . . . and lots of hiking around Lake Wakatipu.

DESTINATION

39

here.) The combination of steep mountains, dark green forests, snowcapped peaks, foaming waterfalls, and fingers of blue fjords make the region one of the most visually stunning temperate areas in the world. Anglers regularly make the pilgrimage to the South Island to fish its clear, uncrowded streams for outsize trout. Wineries are thriving in this former gold mining area. And bungee jumping was conceived here. The region is home to several of the world's most celebrated hiking trails, the Milford and Routeburn Tracks, and lightning-bolt-shaped Lake Wakatipu is popular for jet boaters, kayakers, and anglers.

From its impeccable setting overlooking the lake's northwestern shore, to the lodge's handsome, environmentally sound, and self-sustaining design, no detail has been overlooked. "At the core of my relationship with Chris is the idea that humans are able to evolve our relationship with existence," Damian reflected. "We're born into a state of pure awareness. When we're very young, this allows us to be in a state of wonder with the mundane—a leaf blowing in the wind, rustling grass. We get away from this as we grow older. Yet it's still there, just underneath, unchanged. All we need to do is come home. Eating, enjoying the breeze, and looking at the stars can all help cultivate a return to who we are. Here at Aro Ha, we're stringing together practices to give guests a greater frequency of presence, a peaceful relationship with the moment." To that end, interaction with nature is a large component of the program. There's no Wi-Fi in public areas to help guests break from their technology and be more in the now. A plant-based diet is served to cleanse and heighten clarity—no caffeine, alcohol, or sugar is provided—with many of the vegetables and herbs grown on-site. (Those with trepidations about vegan cooking have not sampled the beet root ravioli with nut cheese filling!)

The typical six-day/five-night stay at Aro Ha is fairly regimented. Damian described a typical day: "At six A.M., guests are awoken by the sound of a Tibetan singing bowl. We meet in the yoga room and are served a morning elixir to start alkalizing the body. After ten minutes of journaling, we lead guests through seventy-five minutes of Hatha yoga, which is followed by breakfast. Then one of our guides will tell us what the day holds, depending on weather. We often leave the site for 3 to 3.5 hours of hiking in world heritage surrounds. There are so many wonderful options in the area, including the Routeburn Track and Greenstone Trail; each day has a dynamic range of intensity levels to choose from. Some areas are moss-drenched, like a scene from *The Hobbit*, others are stark, tussock-covered hills with nary a tree in sight. We get a sense of the area's history, passing old scheelite and gold mines. We invite guests to do mindful walking on trail; many guests fall in love with the silence. Lunch is then served back at the lodge.

"In the early afternoon there's some downtime. Massage is included each full day. Later in the afternoon, guests can attend a variety of classes including hands-on cooking and strength training, and a series we've developed of Aro Ha classes that teach the art of living. We finish with restorative yoga and then dinner." The program includes some potent options like intermittent fasting and taking a vow of silence for a day.

Excellent accommodations and a wisely constructed program are key components of the Aro Ha experience, but the essence of the place is found in the natural surroundings and the manner in which nature helps one connect with the deeper self. Damian shared one such moment: "I was hiking with a group on a day when we were getting heavy snow, which is abnormal. Huge, fluffy flakes were falling rapid fire. I recall walking in this indescribable silence, as the snow was absorbing all of the sound. That silence was amazing."

DAMIAN CHAPARRO is a twelve-year veteran in the health and wellness arena. He is founder and facilitator at the multiaward-winning Aro Ha, consistently ranked in the top-ten wellness retreats globally. He teaches yoga as part of an optimal holistic cleanse, which includes hiking, meditation, massage, and plant-based nutrition. Damian is a Yoga Alliance certified instructor and brand ambassador to Manduka and Lululemon.

If You Go

▶ **Getting There**: Visitors fly into Queenstown, which is served by Air New Zealand (800-262-1234; .airnewzealand.com) and Jetstar (866-397-8170; jetstar.com) via Aukland and Christchurch. From here, it's roughly forty minutes to Aro Ha.

▶ **Best Time to Visit**: December, January, and February signify the austral summer and are fine times to visit, though fairly clement conditions prevail from October to April. Retreats are held at Aro Ha year-round.

▶ **Accommodations**: Aro Ha (+64 34427011; aro-ha.com) offers six-day/five-night retreats, including all classes, excursions, and meals.

DESTINATION

39

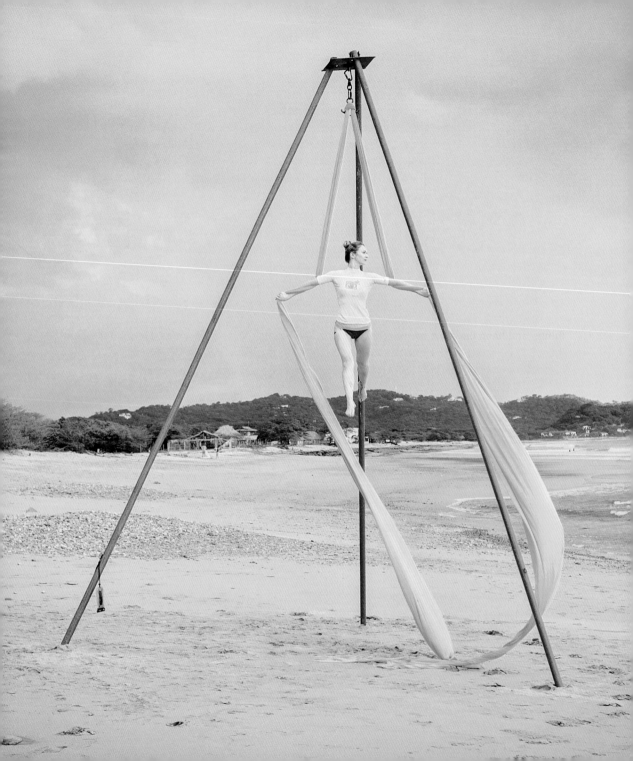

POPOYO

RECOMMENDED BY **Kerri Flannigan**

"I'd been to Costa Rica and Mexico, and I loved the environment, but I wanted to search for something a little different," began Kerri Flannigan. "My background is on the fitness side, and a lot of the yoga retreats you see are more meditation focused, more inward. I wanted a place where we could have that but also do fitness-based workouts, learn new things, and hang the AIR® hammocks. I searched and searched but didn't see anything that fit this. Then I found Magnific Rock in Nicaragua."

Nicaragua sits near the middle of Central America, bordered by Honduras to the north and Costa Rica to the south, with ample coastline along the Caribbean and Pacific. Often called a "surf and yoga playground," the sprawling, wooden retreat center of Magnific Rock is perched on a thirty-meter cliff on the southeastern coast, where emerald rainforest meets the Caribbean. The nearby Popoyo Surf Zone has been called a "miracle" of beach and reef breaks, combining the power of frequent south swells with consistent offshore winds from Lake Nicaragua, attracting surf-seekers and beach-lovers from across the globe. "It's a 2.5-hour drive from the airport down this rocky, dark road, and that's after your long international flights, so you're looking at a total of seven to ten hours to get here, for most people. You're exhausted, you're cranky. And then, as soon as you step out of the cab and onto the property, you're suddenly standing on the side of this gigantic rock. The wind is all over you and you're looking at a 360-degree view of the beach. Everyone is barefoot. It's rustic, it's dirty but, at the same time, so clean. [At that moment] you escape reality and fall into a new kind of culture. It's like a utopia."

With this environment, the Nicaraguan coast has been increasingly playing host to numerous international yoga retreats. Aerial yoga in particular—the hybrid workout that began in 2014, combining Pilates and yoga poses with the anti-gravity benefits of a

OPPOSITE:
A known
paradise for
surfers, Popoyo
beach also
offers yogis a
chance to play
on sea, land,
and air.

hammock—has moved beyond trendy American workout studios and found a home at Magnific Rock. AIR®, a core-focused, high-intensity workout, is an offshoot of aerial yoga founded by Shama Patel. Kerri brings the workout, along with meditation and more-relaxing deep stretch classes, to Magnific Rock's cliffside by hanging silk hammocks at the hotel's topmost studio space, which faces the blue horizon in all directions. "The first time I walked up to the studio, the windows were wide open, and it took me a minute to let it all sink in," Kerri continued. "It was so quiet. All I could hear was the ocean." Posing in your hammock, with the sounds of the waves and the wind, may be the closest some of us indeed will ever get to flying. "We always practice with the windows wide open and the ocean breathing over us," Kerri added. "It's incredibly calming. We've never had a bad sunset."

If meditating and moving in a sky-bound hammock is not enough of a draw, the beach and the jungle have more to show you. Visitors can hike through the jungle, ride on horseback down the beach, and watch sea turtles making their runs to the ocean at nearby Chacocente, one of the largest wildlife refuge and sea turtle reserves in Nicaragua. Then, of course, there are the waves. "It's a surf town, but most people who come here have never done yoga or surfed before," Kerri noted. "I grew up snowboarding, so I thought surfing would be easy. But it wasn't! The teachers are wonderful, though. They get you extremely comfortable doing a pop-up and then take you into the whitewash. It's scary, but so worth it to feel yourself stand up on a board for the first time. It's powerful when you see everyone able to do it. It speaks to the staff. This is a really peaceful place to learn."

Magnific Rock hosts tourists from across the globe and the center has a strong focus on giving back to the community that has so warmly housed them. "On every retreat, we do one community building and beach cleanup day," Kerri observed. "This year we hosted kids from a local school and taught them an AIR® class. You hear of yoga in schools a lot now in the US, but in Nicaragua no one had ever proposed it to them before; we arranged for them to come visit. The first year we got about twenty-two kids. I'm not fluent in Spanish, so our communication was a little broken, but the kids got so excited when we showed them the hammocks. We all sat down and said hello, did some demonstrations, and then let them at it, while working together to make sure they did it safely. They had so much fun. Then we finished with a breathing exercise and headed down to the beach for cleanup."

Political turmoil has been a part of Nicaragua's reputation for the past 150 years, with unrest abetted at times by the United States. However, after the revolutions of the 1970s and '80s, a relative calm settled over the country and crime rates plummeted to lower than any of its neighbors. In 2019, increases in protests over President Ortega's power began to rock the country once again, but this has not stopped the nurturing spaces where locals and visitors alike come to play, reset, and explore. "The goal is to bring [the peace] home with you, to go on vacation and come back feeling refreshed, rather than 'I ate too much,' or 'I felt too busy.' Instead of feeling like you need a vacation from your vacation, you feel inspired, renewed, like you gave something back to yourself, for yourself."

KERRI FLANIGAN is a certified personal trainer, group fitness instructor, and lifelong athlete. After playing Division II lacrosse at Belmont Abbey College, she discovered AIR® and has been with the company AIR® Aerial Fitness since the studio's beginning in 2014. Now the owner of the Charlotte, North Carolina, AIR® location and owner/founder of the GoodRoots Mvmt retreats, Kerri has made it her mission to provide the tools clients need to create a strong foundation through fitness, adventure, challenge, connection, and self-reflection. With a love for travel, fitness, adventure, and relaxation, Kerri's goal is to help all her students experience what it means to truly live in the moment.

If You Go

▶ **Getting There**: Liberia, in Costa Rica, is the closest airport to Popoyo, served by American Airlines (800-433-7300; aa.com) and KLM (800-618-0104; klm.co.uk). A car, shuttle, or bus will take you the 3.5-hour drive to Popoyo.
▶ **Best Time to Visit**: If you plan on surfing, the best swells tend to be from May through December. Popoyo is sunny most of the year with little rain.
▶ **Accommodations**: Magnific Rock (505-8237-7417; magnificrock.com) has rooms and amenities for both yoga and surf getaways. The Popoyo Tourism Board has a great list of other accommodations at popoyo.com.

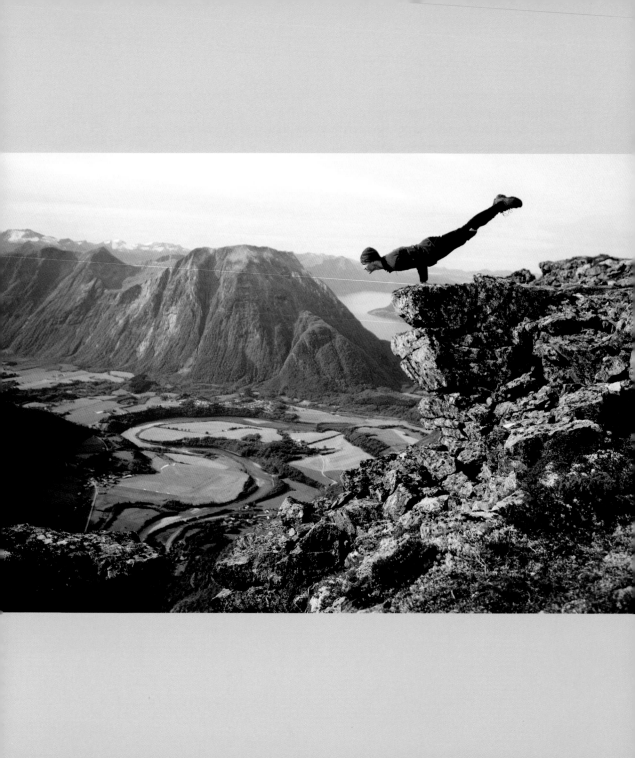

VALDRES

RECOMMENDED BY **Alexander Medin**

One hundred thirty miles north from Oslo, Nøsen Yoga Retreat awaits those who prefer their yoga with a side of sparkling Nordic countryside. Located in Norway's Hemsedal region, often called "the Scandinavian Alps," the area is famous for its ski resorts and fly-fishing opportunities, as well as mountain climbing, biking, and, more recently, yoga. Nøsen's long wooden lodge sits peacefully in a valley surrounded by lush, flowery meadows in the spring and still, white peaks in the winter.

"It's quite an adventure how we got here," reflected Alexander Medin. "I was also working at Back in the Ring, which helps drug addicts get their lives back through yoga, philosophy, and karmic service. I had just taken a group of men to India on a service mission—building shelters, providing community service, studying philosophy—and when we all came back, it came out that a lot of them didn't have any other home to go back to. They needed a place to get out of the networks of bad relations that they knew might pull them back, so I took some of them up to the mountains—to Nøsen—and we began to refurbish this place."

Today, Nøsen is a true haven that goes beyond a simple yoga retreat center. From helping recovering addicts connect to their true selves through yoga and service, to serving as a refugee camp during the 2016 Syrian refugee crisis, the center is a beacon of yogic intention and connection in a landscape of iconic Norwegian beauty. "It took us a while to fix the place up," Alexander continued. "It was so much more work than I imagined when we first got here. Things were falling apart and the roof was leaking. We took off the whole roof and built a new floor with elevated windows. We patched the holes and built new rooms. Now, we have three shalas, a big restaurant and café, and a living room with a fireplace. [The living room] is my favorite place—that's where all the

OPPOSITE:
The epic solitude
of Norway's
countryside
surrounds yogis
at the newly
minted Nøsen
yoga community.

DESTINATION

41

conversation happens. All the rooms on the top floor have a beautiful view of the mountains and the lake and the fields around us. It was finally ours."

As a full-fledged retreat center, Nøsen has become a beacon of yogic philosophy and service in Norway. The lodge can host up to a hundred guests and combines a distinct Norwegian mountain feel with a yogic style and value set. The center offers a spectrum of yoga classes and retreats led by internationally acclaimed teachers. Visiting speakers often include esteemed Tibetan monks, Buddhist scholars, Sufi dance experts, Indian gurus, and respected mystics the world over. "We have acro-yoga, family festivals, meditation retreats, and we host the Norwegian yoga festival every year," reflected Alexander. "Our focus has been on being authentic, making sure there is quality in the yoga we deliver."

A day at the center typically begins around five to six A.M., which, depending on the time of year, means you will be rising into a persistent golden-hour sunrise or a lingering purple twilight. A meditation session gathers the guests, along with a yoga class for all, followed by a healthy vegetarian breakfast, and then a day of asana practice and talks with visiting scholars. "There's always a class in the afternoon, usually on technique, or pranayama, yoga philosophy, or meditation," added Alexander.

Between classes, an outdoor playground awaits. Nøsen is remotely located about twenty miles away from the closest village, and its unique location among almost-5,600-foot (1,700 m) peaks offers mountain-lovers spectacular opportunities to play in some fresh northern air. "Hemsedal is a bit like the area around Aspen," noted Alexander. "Lots of people go walking and trekking into the mountains; cross-country skiing is very popular in winter. There's a beautiful lake right next to us where people swim, canoe, and paddleboard, especially in the summer. Fishing is popular too, of course. In the summertime we have some horses you can rent to ride through the landscape, as well as a farm of goats and chickens that are happy to befriend you. Some people bring their bikes and cycle through the valley and over the hills. There are a lot of activities we try to incorporate. I think the exterior beauty of the area really encourages internal reflection. The goal is to allow people to feel connected and whole while in nature, to feel that untouched serenity from within. This place really facilitates that."

Back at the center, a warm fire, a hot beverage from the café, and a cozy living room encourage conversation between like-minded guests and teachers. In addition to short-term guests, the center welcomes those who wish to stay long term, either as a volunteer or to deepen their yogic practice as a student.

"I had no background in hotel management," concluded Alexander. "I was a traditional ashtanga yoga teacher. The experience here is not about seducing our clients with luxury, but about creating an environment where people feel connected from within and can awaken their inner potential. I didn't know if we could make this work. We had no profit for a long time. But finally, after three years, we started breaking even. It is such an incredible feeling to be able to give people healthy food and good experiences with yoga in a beautiful environment that helps them get in touch with what's really important. That is the most wonderful feeling I can imagine."

R. ALEXANDER MEDIN is a native of Oslo, Norway, where he grew up pursuing many different talents. He became Norwegian champion in boxing at eighteen, but then gave it up for a career as a ballet dancer. He was first introduced to ashtanga yoga in 1995, and it has been part of his daily practice since. After many visits to Mysuru, he was granted a certification to teach ashtanga yoga by K. Pattabhi Jois in 2002—he is one of only thirty-five people to be personally certified by the founder of the style. In 2004, he completed his postgraduate degree in Sanskrit and Indian religions and went on to translate the Yoga Sutras and Bhagavad Gita into Norwegian. In addition to owning Nøsen, he runs the foundation Yoga for Life and launched and continues to run Gangster Yoga and Back in the Ring, helping people who have "fallen out" of society and giving them the opportunity to build themselves up again through a solid yoga practice, heightened sense of responsibility, and social work.

If You Go

▶ **Getting There**: Land at one of Oslo's airports, such as Gardemoen or Torp. From there, take a bus to Fagernes or a train to Gol, where a member of Nøsen's staff can pick you up for a modest fee and complete the forty- to fifty-minute car ride to the center.
▶ **Best Time to Visit**: The area is open year-round. Summer is a great time to fish, canoe, and see the midnight sun. Winter offers ample skiing and snowshoeing opportunities.
▶ **Accommodations**: Nøsen is the only yoga-focused accommodation in the area for many miles, and can be booked at nosenyoga.com or +47 48422888.

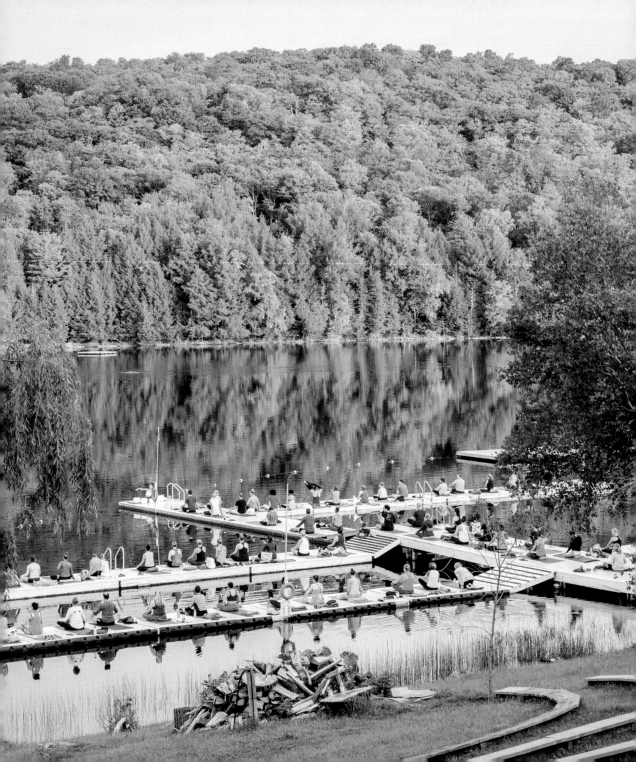

PALMER RAPIDS

RECOMMENDED BY **Sari Nisker-Fox** AND **Jen Birenbaum**

The focus of a yoga retreat. The fun of a summer camp. "I wanted to bring these two worlds together," recalled Jen Birenbaum. "My husband and I co-own Camp Walden, a children's camp about three hours north of Toronto. It's a wide-open natural space where you can jump into a private freshwater lake and feel the trees breathing around you."

In Toronto, Jen met Sari Nisker-Fox, co-owner of Spynga, a prominent Toronto yoga and spin studio. Sari shared her love for the practice and teaching of yoga from the heart, which drew in Jen. Jen completed her first teacher training with Sari at Spynga and, as a result, Spynga Goes to Camp was born.

"It started as a retreat for the studio, held over a weekend in the fall," Jen recalled. "We brought about fifty people the first season, which felt small for a 750-acre property. After running it for two seasons, I dreamed of something bigger, but I was nervous to share that with Sari. Finally, at the end of the second retreat, I blurted out, 'I don't want this to be just for Spynga anymore. I want this to be for everyone.'"

"I was in," Sari said with a laugh. "What's funny is that I was already planning to sell my portion of Spynga but I hadn't even told Jen yet when she said this to me. It was meant to be."

Rebranding the event as the Yoga Weekend, they set out with a goal to demystify the yoga retreat. "It organically became about more than yoga," Sari explained. "We wanted to make it a destination for wellness, with teachers, classes, and human connection. An opportunity to get out of your element, learn about yourself, and try new things. We intentionally did it in September because it's a crazy time with holidays and kids going back to school. So here is a space for *your* summer vacation—just a little weekend to leave the city, reconnect to yourself, nature, and your community."

OPPOSITE:
The premise of
Camp Walden's
Yoga Weekend
is simple:
marry the joys
of summer camp
with the joys
of yoga.

DESTINATION

42

Camp Walden sits tucked behind Ontario's Algonquin Provincial Park, half an hour from the nearest town. Guests stay in rustic cabins with front porches and bunk beds. There are toilets and running water; it's remote, but comfortable. The weekend begins on Friday, as about two hundred people wind their way north from the city. "We congregate in Omni (the theater where the kids put on their talent shows and stage productions during summer camp), and begin our first practice," Jen described. "This is that first moment where everyone is together. It's dark. We have a live deejay and twinkle lights and glow sticks. We take everyone through a mindfulness session and vinyasa flow, encouraging them to let go of anticipation and expectation and to just relax."

Like summer camp, the whole weekend is designed so guests can choose their own adventure. Each block of time offers four or five different workshops or practices. Vision boards are built in the craft workshop. Reiki and massages are offered in the "Farmhouse Spa," the property's original 100-year-old structure. You can water-ski, swim, or paddle out onto the sparkling lake. Cooking classes brew in the kitchen and meals are served communally in the dining hall. Asana flows are held in buildings with floor to ceiling windows, looking out over the forest. Outside, firepits are scattered like stars, awaiting conversation. "We've heard that one of the best feelings about camp is this ability to walk around with no stuff in your pockets," Sari said. "You can just float from one space to another with nothing but a water bottle and maybe a yoga mat."

"Saturday morning, the early birds get up and put on their scarves and gloves and head out to the dock for a first practice," Jen continued. "The lake is like glass. You can see fish jumping and hear birds chirping. As the sun rises, the teachers take everyone through a stillness meditation, then a warming yoga flow. This past year we had a friend play the sound bowls at the end of the dock. During Savasana, she started singing. It was such a magnificent moment. Another morning option is to join a guided meditation on 'the Zen Deck' at the opposite end of the lake."

On Saturday night, "campers" come together on Main Field surrounded by firepits and torches. The deejay plays, and the teachers come together and lead the flow as the sun sets behind the trees. Then campers gather for dinner and have a dance party in the lounge. "Everyone's in their yoga gear," Sari said. "It's like you're dancing in your living room, barefoot, with your friends."

One of the best and most unexpected results of the Yoga Weekend for the two founders was the sense of community that began to sprout. "For most people, this has become less about escaping and more about returning—returning to a community," said Sari. "This isn't a one-off for them. We had one camper tell us, 'You're gonna have to push me in here in my wheelchair when I'm ninety because I'm gonna keep coming!'"

SARI NISKER-FOX is a mama of two girls, a yoga and mindfulness teacher, a speaker, a holistic life and purpose coach, an entrepreneur, and a visionary. She has lived and breathed the wellness and yoga space for over fifteen years in New York City, LA, and Toronto. As a former fitness and yoga studio owner, facilitator of annual yoga teacher trainings, workshops, and classes, Sari has taught and inspired thousands of people. Sari brings mindfulness and self-care practices into different corporations, wellness studios, and homes sharing how living well is possible. As co-creator of the Yoga Weekend retreat and a supporter of annual wellness events in Toronto, Sari's love for building community and inspiring ways to live a present life through movement, mind-set, and purpose is at the core. Learn more about Sari at sarifox.com.

JEN BIRENBAUM is a proud mama of four, creator of hOMe private yoga studio, co-owner of Camp Walden, and co-founder of the Yoga Weekend. This beautiful wellness retreat is not only a passion project for Jen, but also a culmination of her camp experience and love of yoga. Jen is passionate about sharing the practice of yoga. Through her own practice, she has come to embody the importance of having a space to explore and discover oneself. Jen aspires to meet people where they are to support the process of healing and growing. Learn more about Jen at jenbhome.com.

If You Go

▶ **Getting There**: Camp Walden is two to four hours away from several international airports, including Toronto and Montreal, but Ottawa is the closest. From there, rent or catch a ride in a car for the two-hour drive (there is no public transport to Camp Walden).
▶ **Best Time to Visit**: The Yoga Weekend is a yearly event that takes place in early fall, usually in September.
▶ **Accommodations**: You can reserve a spot at camp at theyogaweekend.com.

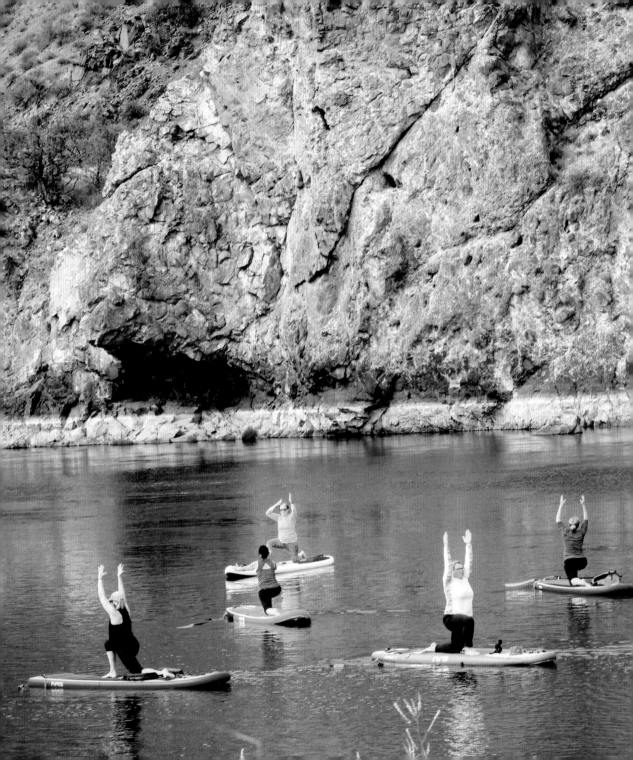

JOHN DAY RIVER

RECOMMENDED BY **Mia Sheppard**

Running over five hundred miles between its three branches in northeastern and central Oregon, the John Day is the third-longest free-flowing river in the United States, and is protected as a "Wild and Scenic River" under the Oregon Scenic Waterway Act. The isolated canyons of the John Day—sometimes called the Grand Canyon of Oregon—provide a majestic backdrop for outdoor enthusiasts and anglers who travel from far and wide to pursue smallmouth bass or steelhead. It's an equally stately setting for practicing yoga . . . on a standup paddleboard!

OPPOSITE: The wild and scenic John Day River provides a stunning backdrop for a one-of-a-kind SUP yoga float trip.

"I've been practicing yoga off and on for twenty-five years," Mia Sheppard began. "It's always something I've tried to incorporate into my daily routine. My husband and I have been guiding anglers on the John Day since 2003. For almost that long, I've had this little dream of assembling a yoga float trip on the river. As outfitters, we always need to diversify and add new offerings to bring new people to the river. Back in 2016, we introduced the option for anglers to float and fish the river on a standup paddleboard instead of a raft or drift boat. The John Day is phenomenal for SUPs—the river is very slow, methodical, with no big rapids. A few years later, I met a yoga instructor in the Columbia Gorge named Amie DiGennaro who'd been doing SUP yoga for several years. I approached her about doing a yoga trip on the John Day, and she was eager to sign on."

No water sport in recent memory has gained momentum as quickly as standup paddleboarding (SUP), where practitioners use a single-bladed paddle to propel an extra-long (and slightly more buoyant than average) surfboard along. SUPs allow the maneuverability and shallow water clearance of kayaks and canoes but afford the paddler a higher vantage point, allowing you to see *below you* as well as around you. The phenomenon appears to have materialized out of nowhere, though the practice dates back to the 1960s, when paddles were used by Hawaiian surf instructors to help newbies get the hang of standing up on a board. The same instructors would paddle themselves around when the surf was flat as a means of staying in shape. It was two surfer/entrepreneurs, Deb and Warren Thomas, however, who brought the first commercially available SUPs to market from their home in Santa Barbara.

SUPs are a good way to get around on the water and tone your core, but do they make good yoga mats—in a river?! "There are a couple key elements to SUP yoga," Mia explained. "First, you need a stable board. We use SUPs that are 36 inches wide, 10½ or 11 feet long, and 5 or 6 inches thick. (The average SUP is 30 to 32 inches wide.) The bigger board provides a very stable platform. Second, you need a calm surface. As mentioned before, the pace of the John Day is slow enough when we go (late June) that it's almost like a lake. We use anchors to keep the board in place. You feel only a very gentle movement from the river, a slight sway back and forth. I find something powerful when I do yoga on the SUP, a connection of my breath to the water and the elements." There are some poses that lend themselves especially well to SUP yoga. "Downward Dog is a great beginner's paddle yoga pose," Mia continued. "It helps you find your balance, connecting you with the slow movement of the board in the water. The Child's Pose is also good on the board. Warrior Poses are a bit trickier. When the sun is out, it's tough to beat Savasana." There are generally two SUP yoga sessions a day during the three-day float. If the weather isn't cooperative, there's always the option of land-based practice.

As is the case for many yoga practices, the path is the goal on a John Day float. The twenty-five-mile excursion takes you past stunning scenery—you'll float by imposing rock formations of vertical basalt, and abandoned cabins of early homesteaders, and will likely spy some of the region's fauna—bighorn sheep, pronghorn antelope, or mule deer on the cliffs, and golden eagles, bald eagles, and pygmy owls on the wing. Several Native American tribes once called the canyons home, including the Northern Paiute. In the course of a float, you may linger at several places to witness remnants of Indian life—pit house foundations with obsidian shrapnel scattered about, petroglyphs (incised rock art), and pictographs (drawn rock art).

"Some people think that you have to stand the whole twenty-five miles," Mia added. "That's not the case at all. You can kneel on the board as you float down, or even sit." When you arrive at the designated camping spot each afternoon, your tent and the dining area are all set up by our professional team. All camping gear is provided." Though you're camping, you'll enjoy excellent meals. Grilled salmon is a favorite, but the chef can easily accommodate any dietary restrictions. Before or after dinner, there's time to take a hike into the canyons or along the river, or relax with a book or glass of wine.

The sublime isolation of a John Day yoga float exquisitely reveals itself on the first evening. "We do a yoga session on the river, surrounded by rim rock," Mia enthused. "It's a coliseum of basalt. All the sounds echo—the birds' calls, the wind, Amie's instructions. As the sun sets, there's alpenglow. The basalt lights up, glistening orange and red. The sky is pink and purple."

MIA SHEPPARD is a lover of wild rivers, world champion spey caster, accomplished guide, conservationist, snowboarder, and mother. In 2003, Mia and her husband purchased Little Creek Outfitters and she started her guiding career on Oregon Rivers. Today she is recognized as one of the world's top female anglers and has used her casting skills to raise over $18,000 for Casting for Recovery. When she isn't on the river, or being a mom, she is working to engage more women and children in the sport of fly-fishing and the outdoors through her company Juniper River Adventures. She currently serves as a commissioner for Travel Oregon (the state's tourism board) and is an ambassador for Simms Fishing, Smith Optics, Airflo, and Keep Fish Wet.

If You Go

▶ **Getting There**: Most visitors fly into Portland, which is served by many major carriers. From there, it's a 2.5-hour drive to Condon, where trips stage.
▶ **Best Time to Visit**: SUP yoga trips on the John Day are generally led in late June or early July, as river flows are ideal at this time. Trips are offered by Little Creek Outfitters (541-419-2105; fly-fishing-guide-oregon.com).
▶ **Accommodations**: On the river, you'll stay in comfortable tents that have cots and pads and delicious camp meals (all diets can be accommodated). Condon, where you'll stay before the trip launches, has two lodging options: Condon Motel (541-384-2181) and the Historic Hotel Condon (541-384-4624; hotelcondon.com).

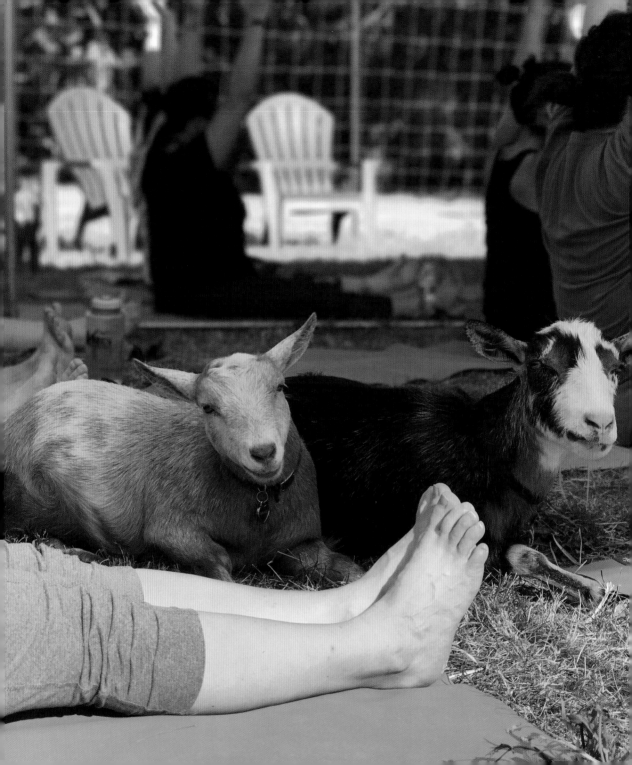

OREGON CITY

RECOMMENDED BY **Lainey Morse**

Pop culture trends come and go. *Game of Thrones*. The Ice Bucket Challenge. Justin Bieber (though "the Biebs" does seem to display a strange half-life). One trend from the late 2010s that's had unlikely staying power is the phenomenon of goat yoga—that is, people practicing yoga in the company of young goats.

"Goats were among the first domesticated animals," observed Lainey Morse, the progenitor of goat yoga. "They've been bred for many years to respond to humans. They like to have fun, they like to play. And they're herd animals. They like to be together. When you come into their barn, you become one of their herd and they like to be by you. Most people have never had any interactions with goats. But when you lay your mat down and these goats come to you and snuggle, it's comforting. When they chew their cud, they go into an almost meditative state. It's oddly relaxing to listen and watch. When you're around them, you take on that energy."

Goat yoga grew out of Lainey's curiosity and affection for the *Capra* genus of mammals. Around the time she was grappling with the double whammy of a divorce and a disease diagnosis, she acquired two baby goats for her small farm in Oregon's southern Willamette Valley—a longtime dream. Walking among the goats after work provided a profound sense of relaxation for Lainey. Soon she felt that keeping this special form of therapy to herself would be unfair, so she began inviting friends to come by for "Goat Happy Hour."

On one occasion, Lainey auctioned off a child's birthday party to raise funds for a local charity. This proved fortuitous, as one mother in attendance asked if she could hold a yoga class with the goats. "That first class—I was there taking pictures—one of the goats jumped up on someone's back as they were doing a pose," Lainey recalled. "Goats are

OPPOSITE:
Goats not only provide an Instagram moment; their presence seems to help yogis reach a more meditative state.

prey animals and they like to be up high to see what's coming, whether that means climbing up on a chair, a table, or a human. I got that shot and posted it online. It went viral pretty quickly, and suddenly the idea of goat yoga was born." (Lainey pointed out that generally it's only the baby and teen goats that will jump up on someone's back. Goat yoga practitioners generally retain Nigerian Dwarf and Pygmy goats as their assistants.)

Original Goat Yoga—Lainey's company—currently has sixteen affiliated locations around the United States. Original Goat Yoga's second Oregon location is in Oregon City, just southeast of Portland. Given "Portlandia's" proclivity for slightly eccentric notions, it's no wonder that goat yoga has thrived here. Indeed, the City of Roses was already home to several intriguing yoga variants, including:

- AcroYoga: As the name implies, this practice combines acrobatics and yoga, and often involves poses balancing atop another practitioner.
- Aerial yoga: Fabric slings enable participants to take their asana practice to new heights.
- Beer yoga: All-levels flow "detox and retox" classes are held at various brewpubs around town, followed by pints.
- Cannabis yoga: Here, participants consume cannabis first and then make their way through (safe!) beginner poses.

There's no set schedule for how goat yoga classes unfold. Instructors are given some latitude in accordance with their preferences. Lainey described the general experience. "If it's a sunny, warm day, people might assemble outside. If the weather's not as good, students will collect in the barn. The teacher might lead students through ten minutes of stretching, and then the goats will come in. Everyone's so excited. As students start to assume poses, the goats might nibble on their mats or nuzzle their shoulders. Some instructors like to do more ground poses, so students are closer to the ground. [Remember that Instagram moment!] Initially, the actual yoga portion of the session was an hour, but since many people coming to a class are doing yoga for the first time, we scaled things back. Now, we usually do a half hour of yoga and then an hour of Goat Happy Hour."

Goat yoga has been a source of great joy for most participants, but not all have responded favorably. "Some animal activists came after me when we started getting publicity," Lainey recalled. "Far-right religious groups accused me of being a cult leader and engaging in satanic worship. Even some members of my family, who are very religious, questioned me." Any negativity, however, has been more than overshadowed by stories like this: "After one class, I had a lady come up with tears in her eyes," Lainey shared. "She'd been the primary caregiver for her husband, who had cancer. She'd almost canceled her ticket to come to Oregon, but her daughter encouraged her to visit. She said that goat yoga was the first time she'd smiled or laughed in months."

Baaa-maste to that sentiment!

LAINEY MORSE hails from Michigan, but she has lived in Oregon since 2006. She has worked in the business development and marketing fields for over twenty years, and has been an award-winning professional photographer. Goat yoga was born when a friend asked if she could lead a class at her farm, No Regrets, in the Willamette Valley. After hundreds of appearances in publications and media outlets including CNN, the *New York Times*, *Time*, *Wall Street Journal*, NPR, BBC, and many more, Lainey found her voice describing how to persevere in the face of adversity, the power of reconnecting with our rural roots, the fulfillment borne of helping others to realize their dreams, and the joy that comes from a goat picking your yoga mat to lie on.

If You Go

▶ **Getting There**: Oregon City is a short ride from the Portland airport, which is served by most major carriers.

▶ **Best Time to Visit**: Goat yoga sessions are offered throughout the year (generally on the weekends) at Beaver Lake Stables. Original Goat Yoga (888-992-4628; goatyoga.net) lists class schedules and other details. Private events are also available at No Regrets Farm & Sanctuary near Albany, Oregon, where goat yoga began.

▶ **Accommodations**: Travel Portland (travelportland.com) highlights the many lodging options around the Rose City, from restored elementary schools to tiny houses. (The website also highlights some of the region's alternative yoga classes.)

DESTINATION

44

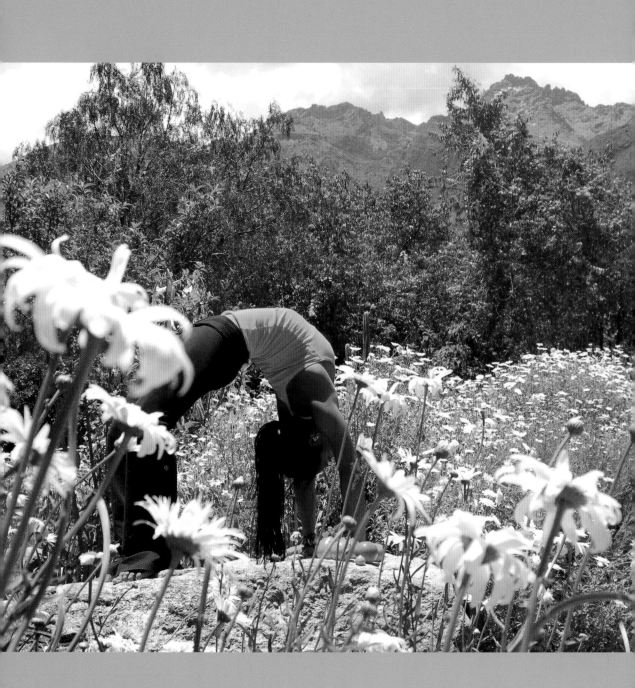

THE SACRED VALLEY

RECOMMENDED BY **Angel Lucia**

"I'm not 100 percent sure what led me to Peru," began Angel Lucia. "I typically don't go in for touristy places, but there's something very inspiring about the culture around Machu Picchu. Everything's coming from the ground and the earth and nature. This is a great place to get tuned into the natural world and let it inform your yoga practice."

The mystical Incan archaeological site of Machu Picchu has been attracting hikers, spiritual seekers, and explorers for hundreds of years. Archaeologists theorize that the Sapa Inca ("god emperor" of the Inca) may have had the city built around 1462 as a vacation retreat. Apparently abandoned a hundred years later, it luckily evaded discovery by Spanish conquistadors during the colonization of South America. The West would not be introduced to the ruined city until American expeditioner Henry Bingham came to Peru in 1911. (Despite the site's occasional nickname, "the Lost City," he found it inhabited by a handful of local farmers, indicating perhaps to the Peruvians it was never lost at all.)

Today, Machu Picchu is on the bucket list of nearly every world traveler, and for good reason. The World Heritage Site will please yogis eager for an experience with deep connections to the earth and who have an unquenchable love of heights. Famed as the site of a very powerful energy vortex (which some believe to be the same force the Incas referred to as "Pachamama"), it is the perfect place to connect to earth energies, but with some caveats. "You can't do yoga right on the rocks," noted Angel. "It's a protected site, often flocking with crowds, and tours must be booked well in advance." However, for yogis in the know, a rich, less-crowded experience awaits just below, in the Sacred Valley.

The Sacred Valley is a green enclave nourished by the Urubamba River at the foot of Machu Picchu. It is resplendent with historical sites and has small towns brimming with

OPPOSITE:
The Sacred Valley
of the Incas below
Machu Picchu
offers magical
gardens and
opportunities to
talk with local
shamans.

DESTINATION

45

201

local culture, space to explore and wander, and abundant flora. Yogis will find themselves warmly greeted at Willka T'ika, a sustainable, culturally responsible wellness retreat center that caters to yogis wishing to connect conscientiously to the landscape.

Founded in 1994, the center features a staff of local Quechua people, loyal yoga teachers, spiritual leaders, an abundant farm-to-table menu, and everything a visitor might need to relax and connect to the mountainscape. "The owner bought the land raw and created the whole center," recalled Angel. "She had a local Quechua shaman walk through the site with her, and he informed her, 'You have a very spiritual space here,' then took the time to educate her about what she should and should not do there."

Willka T'ika boasts numerous yoga shalas and workshops that blend yogic aesthetics and spirituality with Peruvian culture and magic. "There's a huge firepit in the garden, where we do koka leaf readings. Occasionally, shamans come in the evening to visit and give talks. You can learn so much about these elders who are still doing their magic. The shaman we met with spoke only Quechua, but there is a translator to help out. It's an incredible experience to be outside listening to the elders under the insanely bright stars," Angel reflected. "You feel like you're inside of the stars."

In addition to discussions with local leaders, visitors can meander through the meditation gardens representing the seven chakras, each one with flowers, colors, and energies representing the chakras. "The gardens are pure magic," Angel enthused. "They house the most beautiful flowers of every color along with clusters of large crystals. A labyrinth is placed within each garden to ensure you walk in a meditative manner, having time to reflect and feel the earth's energy. There is also an enormous lucuma tree at one end of the garden that has been there for hundreds of years. The local shaman who toured the site instructed the owner to keep it—it has its own special powers, its own energies. Being able to sit under this tree, surrounded in the gardens by all of these amazing plants, crystals, and incredible energy . . . I would go back just for that."

Of course, no trip to the Sacred Valley would be complete without visiting Machu Picchu itself. To reach the site, you can hike over several days, or, for those feeling a bit faint from the high-altitude plunging cliffs, a bus will happily ferry you. "If you get motion sick, you definitely want to take something," Angel cautioned. "And don't look over the edge! The coca leaves help—they really do—but it's still not for the faint of heart or anyone with a fear of heights." Once you reach Machu Picchu, you won't be alone, but there are some special, silent places to be found in the city of rocks. "Our tour guide took us away from the more congested spots—it's great to work with a guide who really knows where to go," Angel advised. "When you step out of these little portals and see the clouds and the valley below, it simply takes your breath away. And, of course, we can't forget to mention the llamas and alpacas wandering around, hopping up and down on different terraces."

ANGEL LUCIA is an ERYT500, RYS200, and YACEP certified yoga teacher and teacher trainer, as well as a licensed massage therapist and certified holistic health counselor. She is the founder of Bindu Yoga Studio in West Palm Beach, Florida, and a former contributor on topics of mindfulness for West Palm Beach's Channel 12 news. Teaching yoga and guiding students deeper into their own mysteries for the past twenty-three years has been her greatest gift. Angel leads retreats in many different countries and has taught in American youth runaway shelters, homeless shelters, and centers for persons recovering from addiction. She has also worked with prominent athletes, political figures, and many high-profile clients. She wants to empower everyone to be their own true guru, and knows that traveling and experiencing different cultures and distant lands can allow us to understand one another better and see how interconnected we all are.

If You Go

▶ **Getting There**: Cusco is the nearest airport, but it is served only by South American carriers. International travelers will have to arrive in Lima and make a connection to Cusco. From there, either hop on a bus or into a collective van for the hour-and-a-half ride to Ollantaytambo. Private tours that include airport transfers and guides to Machu Picchu are also a popular option.

▶ **Best Time to Visit**: May through September are the driest and most popular months. October through December, while slightly rainier, afford fewer crowds.

▶ **Accommodations**: Willka T'ika (willkatika.com; 805-884-1121) is open year-round. Other accommodations in the Sacred Valley can be found with the Peruvian Exports and Tourism Board (peru.travel).

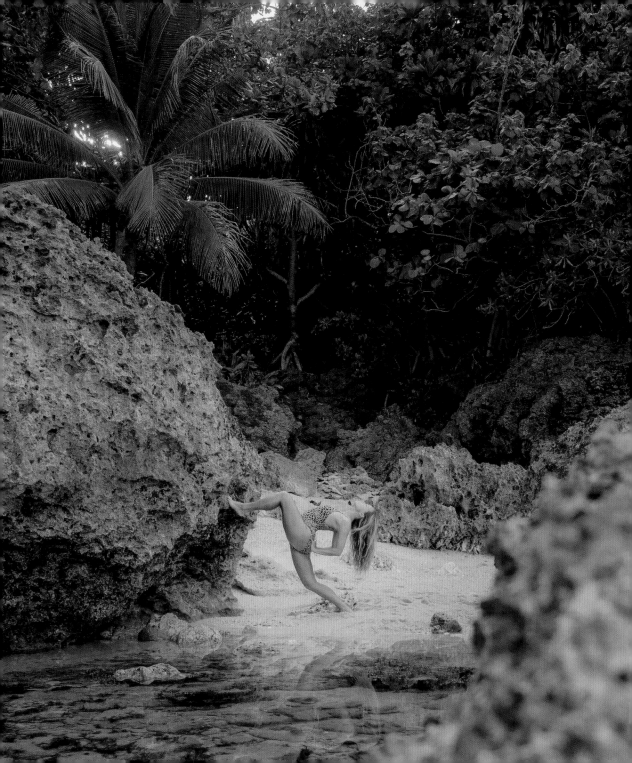

SIARGAO

RECOMMENDED BY Rachel Wainwright

You're not likely to bump into Siargao unless you already know where it is; getting there from abroad involves complicated travel arrangements and long layovers. However, many yogis believe it's this placement off the beaten path that has led to Siargao remaining a pristine paradise. "Literally from the moment I arrived, I began falling in love with this place," began Rachel Wainwright. "It completely took my breath away. The whole island is lapped with turquoise surf waves and clean beaches, and—I've been all over the South Pacific—these are the most beautiful palm trees I have ever seen. The community is extremely friendly. People literally sing in the streets (karaoke is huge here). It is not very expensive or very corporate. It is a place where you can completely connect to nature. It's different from India and Bali, where the yoga culture is rooted in Hinduism. However, the way people live here is very yogic."

Siargao is just one of the 7,107 islands in the Philippines and has spent most of the last thirty years serving as the country's surf capital. "The locals welcome tourists, but they are very aware of the impact civilization can have on nature," Rachel continued. "Eco-consciousness reigns supreme. They have tons of water initiatives, beach cleanup days, and lots of single-use plastic education. And it's not the government that's doing this, it's really the people. They know how precious their island is, and they are striving—and succeeding—at preserving it."

This connection to nature is a big part of why Rachel, having sold her yoga studio in Vancouver, British Columbia, a few years earlier, decided to host an Exhale Yoga retreat at the yoga shala Soultribe, one of a handful of shalas on the island. "Using nature in your practice is very powerful, and this is a wonderful place to connect to the elements," she opined. "You go into the palm tree forest in the afternoon, and the light is beaming through

OPPOSITE:
Siargao is
difficult to get to,
but the unspoiled
island vibe is a
rich reward.

DESTINATION

46

the leaves, you hear birds singing, and you feel the air . . . you are inspired to drop into a deeper place in yourself. And this image, what I'm describing here, this is the whole island, not just one area."

Flawless beaches, azure waters, and feathery palm trees aren't the only thing magical about Siargao. "Cloud 9" break, famous for its massive, hollow tubes, is the setting for the the Siargao Surfing Cup Competition, one of the largest sporting events in the Philippines. "Even if you came here for yoga, and not surfing, many who come here end up learning to get on a board," continued Rachel. "Surfing actually aligns with yoga very well. It's about letting go, connecting with nature, being humble, literally going with the flow. And you have to pay attention and be in the moment, because the minute you don't, you get slapped in the face by a wave!"

Not all currents that run along Siargao's shores end in famously strong breaks, so if surfing's not your thing, there's still a variety of ways to get in the blissfully blue water. "You can paddleboard—the air is so fresh along the channels of the rivers," described Rachel. "You can also scuba way off shore, or snorkel in the reefs right along the beaches. You can parasail, kite-surf, or kayak. Often on a retreat here, we take a boat and go island hopping." Guyam, Duku, and "Naked Island" (named for its barren sandbar appearance rather than its unclad locals) are tiny, uninhabited islands that decorate the horizon, and boats and tours can be chartered for a fun day trip.

Although it seems the "tropical beach of your dreams," according to Rachel, the few yogis that make it out to Siargao go there to do deep internal work to reconnect to their true self and life's purpose. "When people set off on a yoga retreat, it's usually because they've had a bad year. Maybe they lost their job, are going through a divorce, they're feeling directionless, they've lost purpose. Most people aren't here because they are having a good time. So it ends up being way more than a yoga holiday in paradise. When you are far from home, there's no running off and away from anything you're feeling after class, no meter to feed, no kid to feed. You have to focus on yourself; you have no excuses. This can be harder than most people think. Society doesn't often praise the courage you need to let go of things that aren't serving you. But here, we have the space and calm to talk about that, and about how to make the changes to achieve what you need in a way that's non-harmful to others."

Siargao lends itself well to the self-exploratory, life-coaching-style yoga retreat Rachel wanted to produce. "The nature nurtures your nature," she reflected. "You're surrounded and supported by the elements—this is something you can really get in Siargao. We do pranayama breathing with the sunset. We're mainly vegan, serving local produce, but sometimes a fisherman will bring in something they've recently caught. We have a no-cellphone policy at dinner so people can really connect and share and experience the world around them. And the asana practices get to be long. They really serve to open you up. It is so beautiful to practice when you can feel the breeze on your skin, feel your feet on the earth, and then cleanse yourself in the ocean.

"When people arrive, they're like a knitted ball, and each day we unravel another knot . . . and then they start rolling in the direction they want to. It's a beautiful thing to see."

RACHEL WAINWRIGHT is a certified life coach, Yoga Alliance certified yoga teacher, and the founder/owner of Exhale Yoga Retreats. Yoga has given Rachel the tools to meet the inevitable difficulties of life with a measure of acceptance, openness, trust, and love. She believes that with this practice you will attract a healthier, happier, more fulfilling life. Rachel attracts like-hearted people from around the globe to come to paradise to unite a higher frequency of good vibes. Through her yoga classes infused with her life-coaching skills, she inspires profound transformation and seeks to create an empowering sense of connection. Her online classes are featured on Gaia, and the full company of her yoga, Pilates, and Jungle Dance classes can be found at rachelwainwright.com, or find her on Instagram at @yoga.rachel. More information about Rachel's retreats is at exhaleyoga retreats.com and on Instagram at @exhaleyogaretreats.

If You Go

▶ **Getting There**: Visitors fly into Manila then on to Siargao, which is served by Philippine Airlines (800-435-9725; philippineairlines.com) and Cebu Pacific (+632 87020888; cebupacific.com).

▶ **Best Time to Visit**: It's relatively dry between March and November, while the rest of the year is subject to monsoon rains. September to November sees the most surfing events.

▶ **Accommodations**: The Soultribe surf and yoga lodge (soultribebeachretreat.com) can accommodate visiting yogis.

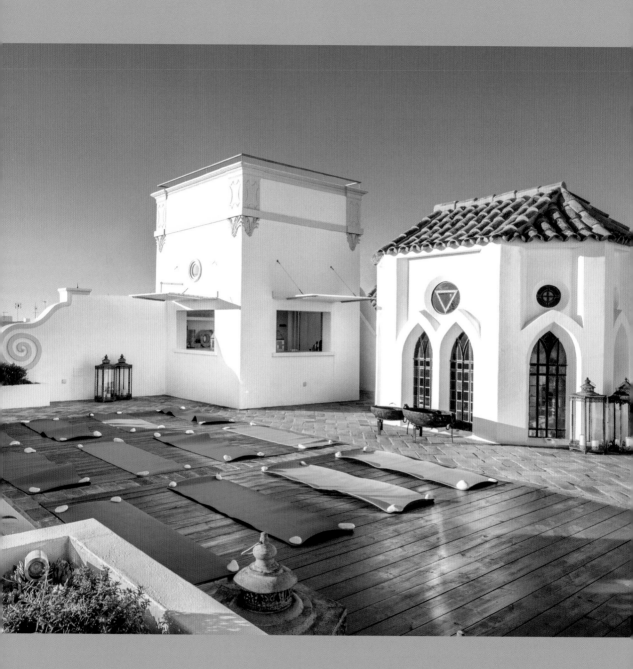

OLHÃO

RECOMMENDED BY **Tara Donovan**

The crystal-clear waters, sun-colored cliffs, and faded white arches of Portugal's south-western coast are hardly a secret, at least to most European vacationers seeking a North African vibe without having to cross the Mediterranean. "The Brits have dominated the development of the western Algarve," reflected Tara Donovan. "It's hard to explain how different, culturally, the west side of the region is from the east. The west, the area right on the water with the beaches, has been heavily developed and now includes many five-star resorts and gated communities, manicured to within an inch of their lives and with very little connection to traditional Portuguese culture."

For those less into high-end golf courses but still seeking an authentic, uniquely Portuguese experience, Tara advises that you drive half an hour east. "The fishing town of Olhão, sheltered by the hills of the eastern Algarve, is technically still on the coast," she described, "but it doesn't have its own beach. And in some ways, I think that is what has saved it from development. It still has this authentic, North African medina feel."

Olhão is the site of Casa Fuzetta, one of Portugal's premier yoga retreat destinations, booking some of the UK's and the world's most prominent yogis up to two years in advance. The house itself is the combination of three buildings, a multiroomed mansion in the style of Portuguese minimalism, complete with towering white walls, geometric brick floors, high ceilings, great halls, breezy terraces, and a modern rooftop pool.

Tara's husband Jonathan stumbled upon this house on his first visit to Olhão in May 2013. The house was derelict but there was this inner courtyard and a chapel-like structure on the roof. When Jonathan took Tara back at the end of September 2013, they both felt the pull of the house. "Everybody told us it would take at least four years for planning permissions and renovations, but we ended up getting it all together in two

OPPOSITE:
Portugal's
Eastern Algarve
retains its old-
world charm,
especially
in the fishing
village of Olhão.

DESTINATION

47

years. A planner with the local government told us, 'You must have a guardian angel for this project. This is unheard of.'"

Tara and Jonathan named the final house after its principal previous owner, local hero Dr. Carlos Fuzeta. "During the renovations," Tara continued, "we came to learn that he was not just a lawyer and philosopher, but a very spiritual person as well. He was very interested in esoteric thinking and probably a freemason. However, he lived in a very conservative, Catholic Portugal. We suspect he had to keep his interests underground. Nevertheless, he inspired a very special energy within the house, and we have sought to recognize and build upon that. Indeed, it is rare for visitors not to remark on how the house feels. In our renovations of the house, we recognized a chakra system—for example, the courtyard space is the heart of the house, and the meditation space holds the crown chakra energy. The meditation room has a chapel-like structure, with stained glass windows, which we restored thanks to a retired local Dutch artist who used to renovate the stained glass windows of cathedrals in Northern Europe. When you walk into the meditation space, there is a stillness and peace that is breathtaking. Fundamentally, this is what we connected with on our first visit and why we bought the space and continue in our role of guardian."

The house continues to grow strong from the energy of numerous yogis who practice morning asanas on the rooftop terrace, or take a golden afternoon dive into the rooftop pool, or share meals in the great hall.

Some might raise their eyebrows at the idea of a yoga retreat in the middle of a city center, but in fact, many guests find it to be a welcome change from more remote retreat settings. "When we first started, we heard [several teachers say that they preferred to do their retreats out in nature]. However, retreat leaders and guests soon started to open up about the fact that the guests wanted more free time to go out and explore and, ideally, be able to do so without needing to hire a car or other complications. As Casa Fuzetta is literally in the heart of the old town, everything is within walking distance and yet also deeply peaceful," reflected Tara.

In Olhão, adventures can include touring the old city, meeting artists in the downtown markets, savoring the booming foodie scene, or island hopping. "We have these amazing markets on the waterfront, full of fruits and vegetables and the best fish in the region. There's a thriving, down-to-earth, rough, and raw vibe that's being generated out here. It's not glitzy; it's very authentic, very real. The community is a mix of a Portuguese fishing town, visitors, and a blossoming creative scene, including some renowned international artists," described Tara.

No tour of the Algarve would be complete without getting out on the water. "You can take a ferry or a river taxi from Olhão, and you'll see there are 37 miles (60 km) of islands just off the coast. It's the only place in Portugal where these types of islands exist. The way they look, you'd think you were in the Maldives. They are empty. I think they must be the only islands in Europe so deserted during the summer. It is absolute magic."

TARA DONOVAN has been a UK-based lawyer, businesswoman, and corporate board advisor for over twenty-five years. She is also the co-owner and renovator of Casa Fuzetta, along with her husband Jonathan Tod, author of *A Starter's Guide to the Meaning of Life*. Tara and Jonathan have been thrilled to host events like "Heal the Healers" and to lead a series of pilgrimages exploring the beauty, history, and energy centers of Portugal. They are delighted to have created a space where some of the world's most prominent yoga teachers, and others interested in exploring spiritual and wisdom traditions, wish to invite their students. Tara is passionate about preserving and sharing the wonders of Olhão. When she's not in Portugal, she lives in London with her husband and two children, William and Daisy.

If You Go

▶ **Getting There**: Faro is the nearest airport to Olhão. It is served by Ryanair (ryanair.com) from most European cities and TAP Air Portugal (800-221-7370; flytap.com) from Lisbon. From either Lisbon or Faro, you can catch a train to Olhão or rent a car for the journey.

▶ **Best Time to Visit**: July to September are the warmest months, so the water temperatures will be the most ideal. However, avoid August if you don't like crowds, as most Europeans take their vacations at that time.

▶ **Accommodations**: Casa Fuzetta books up months in advance, and all offerings are bookable at casafuzetta.com. The Algarve Tourism Board also lists accommodations throughout the region at visitalgarve.pt.

DESTINATION

47

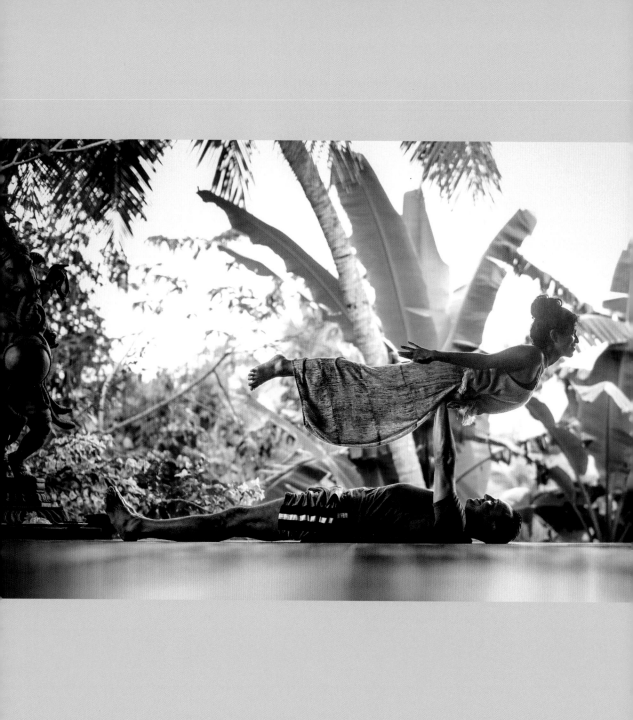

UNAWATUNA

RECOMMENDED BY **Alice Maisetti**

"The first thing that hits you in Sri Lanka is the heat," began Alice Maisetti. "It's a wave of tropical weather. The people are very chill, a mix of local surf teachers and the people who have come to do yoga. It's also very safe. I'm a woman traveling alone and I feel very comfortable."

Sri Lanka, the jewel-shaped island just off India's southeastern coast, has been sighted as an up-and-coming yoga retreat destination for the last ten or so years, fueled by relatively unspoiled and uncrowded beaches and a reputation of safety and hospitality toward tourists. Its name derives from the Sanskrit words *sri* ("venerable") and *lanka* ("island"), and is mentioned in the ancient Indian epics Mahabharata and the Ramayana. A largely Buddhist nation, Sri Lanka boasts a rich history of yoga nearly equal to its Hindu neighbor, dating back to the Vedic period. Countless gurus and mystics have sought refuge or taught here. In the nineteenth century, Mahāvatār Bābājī, the guru famous for bringing kriya yoga from its ancient roots into the modern era, was initiated into the tradition by his masters on this island.

"The yoga scene here is extremely developed," continued Alice. "In south Sri Lanka by the coast, I couldn't even count how many yoga studios and basecamps there are. They blend easily with each other and with various offerings focused on health; there's a very holistic approach to living here."

On the southwestern coast, the popular beach town of Unawatuna has become a hub for foreigners. Famous for its bright coral reefs, palm-lined beaches, surfers coasting the jewel-toned waters of Galle Harbor, and the hippest nightlife on the whole island, it's not hard to see why. "The high season is in early spring," Alice described. "The waves are the best, and the weather is the best. It can be touristy. If you don't like that, you'll find fewer

OPPOSITE:
Sri Lanka has a rich lineage of yogic philosophy and all the natural wonders of a tropical island.

DESTINATION

48

213

people on the island's eastern coast. But it's so worth it here in the southwest. You have these amazing jungle beaches just bursting with green, and the sunsets are something incredible. I can't even explain how lovely they are. Honestly, that's the thing I would recommend: Just go to a beach, literally any beach, at sunset, and wait. You can do some yoga by yourself, and some meditation, and it feels so good. It's like a miracle happening every night."

Sri Lanka is known for its karma yoga, bhakti yoga, jnana yoga, and raja yoga, although today, yoga retreats of numerous lineages abound along both the coast and the jungle interior. "In Unawatuna, there is a yoga center called Sri Yoga Shala about a mile into the jungle from the beach," Alice recalled. "It's owned by a wonderful and friendly Sri Lankan family, and they made this incredible place, just overflowing with green. There's a pool, like a surface of glass, sitting in the middle of the jungle and a big wooden shala with no windows. You can just soak up all the colors and the sounds of what's around you.

"And there are so many animals here! One time I was filming in the forest for an online class on meditation, and I heard something walking behind me. Finally, I had to look, and there was this monkey just walking behind my back, moving slowly, and eating a banana. The animals are very used to people here, so they can get quite close. I've also seen beautiful sea turtles giving birth. They emerge out of the sea and slowly walk on the sand to deliver their eggs. Sometimes, local poachers will sneak in and take the eggs to sell or eat, but another group of locals watches over the eggs to protect them, even digging them up and hiding them, until they hatch and the turtles are big enough to return to the sea. Sometimes when you're swimming in the ocean, you'll see a little turtle head pop up and then go back into the sea."

Inland from the beach, Sri Lanka's palm trees give way to thick jungle vines and rainforest canopies so dense they make their own clouds. The Sinharaja Forest Reserve, a UNESCO World Heritage Site just a few hours' drive inland from the coast, was recently quadrupled in size by the Sri Lankan government due to its important role in hosting a variety of endangered species. "The vibe is completely different in the jungle than on the beach," reflected Alice. "Honestly, you feel like you're in the middle of nowhere, surrounded by nature. People live there, of course, but you can have so many moments where it's just you and the forest. Then, randomly, there will be life. One night, we were driving down this road in the jungle—it was very, very dark—and then, all of a sudden, there was this little stand with music and fairy lights around—and they were serving food. We stopped and said hello, had some *aappa*—little wheat bowls with eggs—and then kept going. This is a normal kind of thing."

"I am in love with this place. Everyone should come here."

ALICE MAISETTI began training in competitive gymnastics at ten years old in Italy, winning several awards and recognitions. Through the years, she has gone on to learn several styles of yoga in India, including advanced practice of asana and movements, as well as pranayama and breathwork. After having lived and taught for seven years in London, she is currently traveling the world to learn from international masters and teach in a variety of shalas. She teaches online classes on YouTube and also contributes to several projects in yoga media, including coaching, retreat organization, and workshops.

If You Go

▶ **Getting There**: Bandaranaike International Airport in Katunayaka is Sri Lanka's only international airport and is served primarily by Sri Lankan Airlines (srilankan.com; +94 117771979). From there, a bus or taxi can take you the few hours by road to Unawatuna and the coast.

▶ **Best Time to Visit**: October to March offer the calmest weather, though temperatures are a fairly constant 80 degrees Fahrenheit year-round. The area is hit hard by the Yale monsoon season from April to September.

▶ **Accommodations**: Sri Yoga Shala (sriyogashala.com; +94 765691672) is the biggest yoga shala in Unawatuna, but smaller hotels, bungalows, and hostels are easily bookable ahead of time or on arrival. A great list is available at srilanka.travel.

48

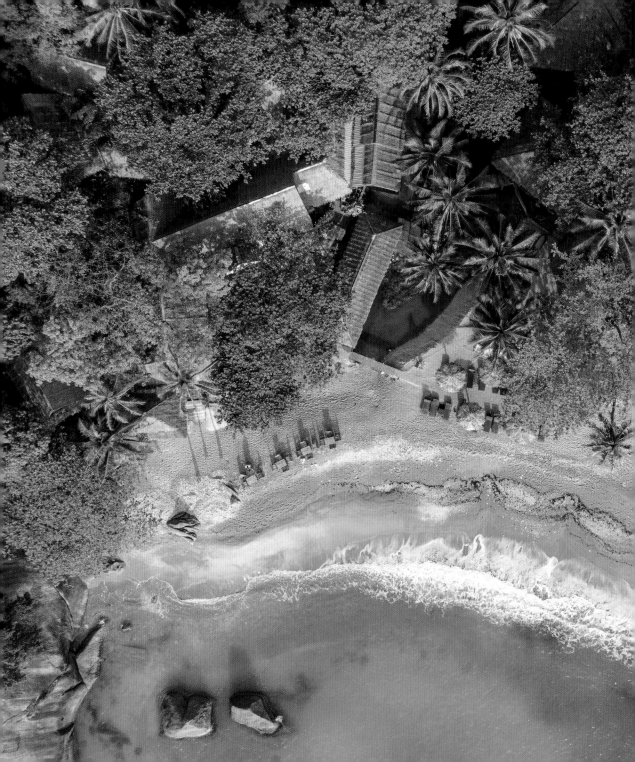

KOH PHANGAN

RECOMMENDED BY **Mike Doyle**

Thailand is no stranger to traveling yogis. The South Asian country, often known as the "land of smiles," is famous for its delicious and affordable vegetarian food, *sabai sabai* ("carefree") hospitality, and a seemingly endless coastline of white sand beaches, perfect turquoise water, and swaying coconut trees. Although largely a Buddhist country, there exists a strong undercurrent of Hinduism as well (Brahmins are known to give blessings before major undertakings, from the beginning of film productions, to the king's coronation). Taoism is also present, thanks to many refugees from China. This philosophical heritage, paired with all the earthly ingredients of a quintessential tropical vacation, comes together in Thailand to create a deeply welcoming environment to practice the union of body and mind. It's no surprise that numerous internationally acclaimed yoga teachers have become expats here, building communities and opening studios throughout the mainland.

OPPOSITE: Thailand is famous for its brilliant blue beaches and alternative healing communes established decades ago.

Offshore, however, is home to even bigger treats. Scattered like emeralds dropped into the bright blue sea, hundreds of small islands lie in the Gulf of Thailand—private, lush, and away from the bustling cities. Although the island of Koh Phangan is known to some for its burgeoning rave scene (epitomized in its "Full Moon Parties"), another side of the island follows the music of a different, slower drum.

"The owners founded the Sanctuary after driving a bus from England to Thailand," reflected Mike Doyle. "On the way, they had stopped at Pune, India (the home of Iyengar yoga), and learned about all these new healing therapies from a few different gurus. Eventually, they got to Thailand, lived here for a few years, and took in everything. And then they started to build. It began with a small beachfront restaurant, a dorm room, and a single yoga hall. This was a long time ago. Yoga and reiki were still very fringe. At the time, the

Christian church was telling people that yoga was bad for spiritual health. We were planting seeds of alternative wellness and growth while trying to keep a low profile and stay hidden."

Located on a remote beach, arrival at the aptly named Sanctuary requires a one-hour ride down a 4×4 mountain track, or a boat ride that cuts you off from the mainland. "Once people get here, they tend to not want to leave," Mike described. "We have three beaches on our bay. Hikes all around. The jungle is safe and warm. I first came here in 1991. I was told there was an alternative healing center opening, that it was on a remote beach on an island, and I was invited to the opening party. We had to climb over the mountain, which took two hours, and we then arrived on a beautiful white sand beach with calm seas and palm trees waving in the wind. I felt like I had stepped through some spiritual membrane, and knew instantly that my life had changed forever. It is different from anything else in Thailand."

The Sanctuary has become an international R&R beacon for both freshly initiated and deeply seasoned yogis. "There's so much going on here it's hard to describe," said Mike. "Yoga used to be the main draw, but now it's more of a foundation for all we do. A lot of people come here for our cleansing detox and wellness programs, while others are just here for an unstructured healthy vacation. We do get some celebrities but nobody really cares, and that's what's great. It's about who you are in the moment here, not who you are out there. People can just come here and be themselves."

An average day might include watching the sunrise on the sea, perhaps with a guided meditation or chi gong, followed by a yoga flow at eight A.M. Breakfast could be home-made yogurt and freshly baked granola, or an item from the raw cleansing menu featuring the jungle's bounty of mangosteen, bananas, coconut, and pineapple. "These days we have a number of digital nomads," noted Mike. More outdoorsy vacationers might spend the rest of the day snorkeling in the calm, turquoise waters of Haad Tien Bay that folds around the resort, or hiking into the hills among the palm and banana trees. Others might visit our treehouse spa or tropical wellness center and sample treats from the healing menu, which includes, of course, Thai massage, as well as Lanna Tok Sen—also known as 'Thai tapping,' where parts of the body are tapped with a mallet and a wooden wedge, activating the energy lines of the body.

"Every week, we also offer a selection of daily mini-workshops, which could be creative writing, astrology, introduction to Ayurveda, or bodywork," explained Mike. "We try to keep an informed atmosphere, where you can learn more about something you knew nothing about before and perhaps find a wellness modality that resonates with you and can go with you on your life's journey. On occasions, the work of Byron Katie and other renowned therapists are made available in workshops, which helps you catch up with yourself through learning what kind of internal work you need to focus on. Two evenings per week, we light more than a hundred candles in the main Buddha hall and practice yin yoga together with a large, golden buddha illuminated by candlelight. It's a very relaxing slow, deep, and calming practice.

"My favorite thing to do is sit in a hammock in the restaurant that overlooks the beach," Mike confided. "I love seeing someone come off the boat with their shoulders hunched up from the day-to-day challenges of life, looking uncertain why they're here, then seeing that same person a few days later with their step light and their demeanor open, and making new friends. There are few places on the planet where you can catch up with yourself and make connections like this."

MICHAEL DOYLE is a retired nurse and an international traveler, and has been "Captain of the Ship" of the Sanctuary since 1998. After working as a nurse and project manager in Australia, Saudi Arabia, and Borneo, Ireland-born Michael came to Thailand in 1991 and could not imagine leaving. He has spent the last twenty-two years guiding the Sanctuary in its offerings of holistic health and wellness, built on the solid foundation of yoga.

If You Go

▶ **Getting There**: The nearest airport to Koh Phangan is Koh Samui, which has frequent flights from Bangkok and Phuket on Bangkok Airways (+66 22706699; bangkokair.com). From the airport take a taxi or bus to the ferry pier, where you can catch one of three ferries a day from Koh Samui's Big Buddha pier to Haad Rin.

▶ **Best Time to Visit**: The main tourist season is from December to March, which is also the dry season. October and November see drenching monsoon rains, although the hot summer often gets showers, as well.

▶ **Accommodations**: The Sanctuary is bookable at thesanctuarythailand.com, and Thailand's Tourism Authority also lists accommodations across the island at tourismthailand.com.

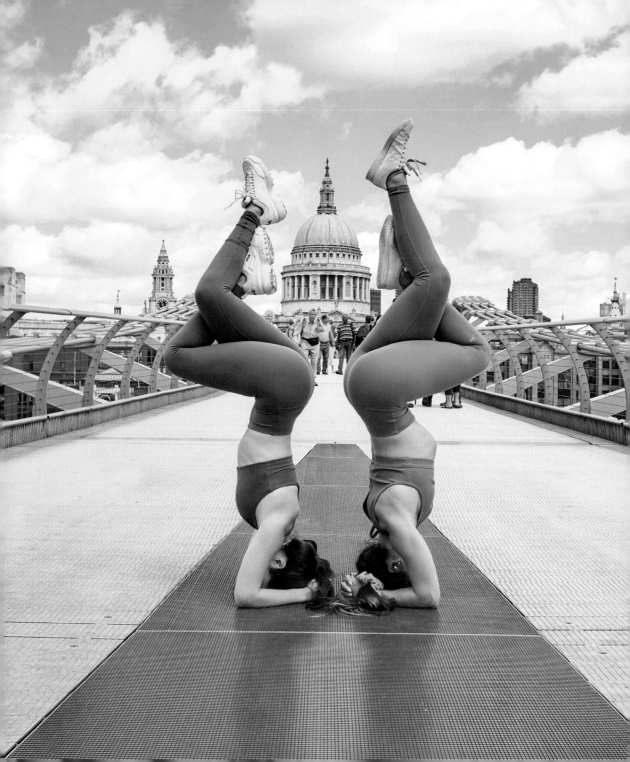

LONDON

RECOMMENDED BY **Stewart Gilchrist**

London, the European culture icon famous for double-decker buses, charming pubs, foggy nights, and Gothic architecture, has rapidly become one of the yoga capitals of the world. Of course, Londoners first encountered yoga via tales from British colonial soldiers in India, wherein devout practitioners were often characterized as madmen. It wasn't until the 1960s, when the Beatles visited Rishikesh with their guru, Maharishi Mahesh, that yoga gained traction in the London counterculture, eventually bubbling up to the mainstream as the influences of ashtanga and Iyengar took the West by storm. Today yoga is an ordinary piece of daily life for the city of nine million; it's estimated that one in four Londoners in their twenties hit the mat at least once a week.

There are far too many internationally revered teachers and beloved shalas in the Swinging City to name in one place. However, Ashtanga Yoga Shala (also known as AYL, or more often, "Dharma Shala") is considered by many to be *the* ashtanga shala in the country, if not the world, second only to the Jois family studios in Mysuru. Although, if you blink while walking down Drummond Street, you might miss it. "It is a really small shala, situated on a small road," described Stewart Gilchrist. "Hamish—one of the most qualified and experienced ashtanga teachers in the world—founded the Drummond Street place and set up Dharma Shala there. The neighborhood has a history of being famous for proper South Indian food, so it felt like a natural place to put it."

The interior of the famous shala is remarkably humble compared to its goliath reputation, with room for only eighteen mats. "It's an innocuous five-by-seven-feet room with paint peeling off the wall and sweat in the air. Maybe a picture of Ganesha. That's it," described Stewart. "But by three A.M. each day, people are outside, queuing up. Hundreds of people pass through the doors in a day. People come in and rotate

OPPOSITE: London challenges yogis who seek out nature to consider how skyscrapers and streets can also be a natural habitat.

221

DESTINATION

50

through the rooms. No one talks; it's Mysuru style, so everyone is doing their own pace. There are no mirrors or music. No heat—all the heat comes from the people. It's just sweat and silence and breathing."

London, like most internationally renowned cities, is known for many things, but peace and solitude are not among them. This can feel to some like a contradiction of yogic aspirations, but for others, this is the point. "People often ask me why I don't go into nature for yoga—why I stay in a city," said Stewart. "London is smog and pollution; it's not pretty, not eco-friendly, and the air quality is the worst in Europe. But concrete and high-rises, skyscrapers and sidewalks, cycling through busy traffic—that is my nature. Yes, some teachers say you should practice outside under the bodhi tree on the skin of a tiger. But there aren't many bodhi trees and tiger skins in London. I spend my life on the freeways; I'm a bike courier.

"The old saying is 'Yoga is 99 percent off the mat'—that your practice doesn't take place in an ashram, it takes place when you're walking about on the street, going to get your children, at university, picking up something from the store. Yoga is something you do in your daily life, not something you do on a mat that you got from Whole Foods made of eco-friendly material. It's something you do when you're with your family, in bed with your lover, on the train, waiting for a bus. The main place to do yoga is in the world. The city of London is a great place for this."

When you're not refining your practice on the streets or in Dharma Shala, London's sheer size affords access to studios in virtually every lineage, plus more than a few unexpected offerings. These include paddleboard yoga in Paddington Basin and vinyasa flow classes in inflatable, bouncy "hotpods," womb-like structures that surround you in 360 degrees of warmth in three locations across the city.

"London is a hive of modern yoga now," continued Stewart. "It's in the fabric of it. One thing visitors should really know is that London is not part of the UK. It didn't vote for Brexit, nor Boris Johnson, nor any of this misogynist, white supremacy stuff that's coming up. It's a true multicultural capital of the world. Where I live in East London, there are forty-two languages spoken and fifty to sixty countries represented within a mile. People in the yoga classes here are from everywhere. And they're all speaking the same language: yoga. That's why I teach here. You can't replicate it."

The moments of yogic bliss to be had in such a bustling city can be quite profound, enough to permanently change your life and alter your being. "At Dharma Shala,

I remember coming out of Savasana and walking out of the studio at 7:30 A.M. as the sun was rising right down the end of Drummond Street. I was watching the sun and had this feeling like I had just peaked on LSD, where everything feels perfect in the whole universe. Before yoga, I'd never managed to experience that feeling without drugs. And listen, Scottish people don't take drugs just one night. We get our hands on something and we just do it for five days in a row. I visited Alfred Hoffman in Switzerland and took LSD straight from the source. But, at Dharma Shala, that was the first time I realized, after I had stopped taking drugs, that a feeling can be this good. And it was all produced in that one little room."

STEWART GILCHRIST is one of London's most sought-after yoga teachers, known for his challenging, innovative classes and potent humor. Originally from Scotland, after working as a teacher and completing his legal studies, Stewart entered the yoga world when a back accident made him reassess his body. He rehabilitated himself through intensive ashtanga yoga, eventually becoming a jivamukti yoga teacher through David Life and Sharon Gannon's instruction. As his practice and knowledge flourished, so did his teaching style, eventually morphing into the energetic flow of Yogasana. He is a registered senior teacher with Yoga Alliance and leads annual retreats in India. Stewart's spiritual journey led him to train all over the world, with teachers who have had a profound effect on his unique style of teaching, including Sabel Thiam, Jennifer Dale, Hamish Hendry, Swami Nirmalananda, and K. Pattabhi Jois.

If You Go

▶ **Getting There**: London is served (via Heathrow and Gatwick) by almost all international carriers.

▶ **Best Time to Visit**: London has a fairly temperate climate, although winter brings frequent rains and summer attracts the highest number of tourists.

▶ **Accommodations**: Hotels, hostels, and homestays are available throughout the city. The Wesley Euston (+44 2073800001; thewesley.co.uk) and Studios2Let (+44 2071216200; serviced.studios2let.com) are just around the corner from Dharma Shala.

Library of Congress Control Number: 2021932565
ISBN: 978-1-4197-5037-3
eISBN: 978-1-64700-475-0

Photography credits: Page(s) 2: © Thomas Klepl; 8: © Tony Felgueiras; 10: © Tom Tietz/Alamy Stock Photo; 12: © Ashley Drody; 16: © Siddharth Saji (Pilfered Tales); 18: © Ben Giardi/Alamy Stock Photo; 22: © Fairmont Chateau Lake Louise; 26: © Liz Gifford/www.lizgifford.com/yoga; 30: © Jen Judge/Aurora Photos; 34: © Chris Daile/Humming Puppy Studio; 38: © Danny Wald; 44: © Tourismusverband St. Anton am Arlberg/ Patrick Bätz; 48: © Yashoda; 52: © David van Driessche; 56: © Jacobus van Heerden; 60: © Kris Krüg; 64: © Jessical Rihal; 68: © Rob Hammer/Alamy Stock Photo; 72: © OwlandBear.org; 76: © Samuel Henderson; 80: © Mount Madonna; 84: © Hariharalaya; 88: © Sasha Juliard; 92: © Red Rocks Amphitheatre/Denver Arts & Venues; 96: © Ashley Drody; 100: © Fritz Grimm; 104: © Anthony Emerson/Stockimo/Alamy Stock Photo; 108: © The Yoga Forest Team; 114: © Hawaii Island Retreat Center; 118: © Samuel Henderson; 122: © Ashley Drody; 126: © Justyna Jaworska; 130: © Atharva Tulsi/Unsplash; 134: © Ananda in the Himalayas; 138: © Ashley Drody; 142: © Roberta Giaccherini; 147: © Lucie Wicker/Cavan Images; 152: © Kripalu Center; 156 : © Westend61 GmbH/Alamy Stock Photo; 160: © Zane Williams Photography: www.zanewilliamsphotography.com; 164: © @spikecrs/Surf Berbere; 168: © Sébastien Goldberg/Unsplash; 172: © Anna Dudko | Dreamstime.com; 176: © C. Stoddart; 180: © Kathryn Moore; 184: © Fartein Rudjord; 188: © Mirza Noormohamed; 192: © Mia Sheppard/Little Creek Outfitters; 196: © Lainey Morse/Goat Yoga; 200: © Willka T'ika; 204: © Jules SeaMan, Exhale Yoga Retreats Photographer; 208: © Garrett Walsh of Algarve Photography; 212: © Sanjin Kastellan; 216: © The Sanctuary; 220: © Alfio Sambataro/Alamy Stock Photo

Jacket © 2021 Abrams

Editor: Elizabeth Broussard
Designer: Anna Christian
Production Manager: Larry Pekarek

This book was composed in Interstate, Scala, and Village.

Printed in Thailand
1 3 5 7 9 10 8 6 4 2

Abrams Image books are available at special discounts when purchased in quantity for premiums and promotions as well as fundraising or educational use. Special editions can also be created to specification. For details, contact specialsales@abramsbooks.com or the address below.

Abrams Image® is a registered trademark of Harry N. Abrams, Inc.

ABRAMS The Art of Books
195 Broadway, New York, NY 10007 ·
abramsbooks.com